MENTAL ILLNESSES AND TREATMENTS

THERAPEUTIC TREATMENTS FOR VULNERABLE POPULATIONS

A TRAINING WORKBOOK

MENTAL ILLNESSES AND TREATMENTS

Additional books in this series can be found on Nova's website
under the Series tab.

Additional e-books in this series can be found on Nova's website
under the e-book tab.

MENTAL ILLNESSES AND TREATMENTS

THERAPEUTIC TREATMENTS FOR VULNERABLE POPULATIONS

A TRAINING WORKBOOK

GRAHAM DANZER

nova publishers
New York

For permission to use material from this book please contact us:
Telephone 631-231-7269; Fax 631-231-8175
Web Site: http://www.novapublishers.com

Library of Congress Cataloging-in-Publication Data

ISBN: 978-1-63117-385-1

Published by Nova Science Publishers, Inc. † New York

I want to acknowledge the faculty at

The Sanville Institute in Berkeley, California

For helping me grow as a professional and as a person

Special Thanks to Dr. Fang-Pei Chen,

Columbia University School of Social Work

CONTENTS

Chapter 1

INTRODUCTION

The mental health care disparity among racial and ethnic minorities is an ongoing social problem that is deserving of national priority (Mental Health America, 2012). Asian Americans are one of the fastest growing populations in the United States and are speculated to have mental illness rates that are comparable to national averages, though are disproportionately underserved due to language barriers and stigma associated with seeking *Western mental health care* (Council of National Psychological Associations for the Advancement of Ethnic Minority Interests, 2003; Office of Minority Mental Health, 2009). African-Americans are often misdiagnosed with having severe mental illnesses, tend to enter mental health treatment in later stages of illness development, are disproportionately admitted to state hospitals, and often discontinue treatment services after the initial session (Council of National Psychological Associations for the Advancement of Ethnic Minority Interests, 2003; Parham et al., 2003). Latino populations in America are growing at faster rates than what was once projected, usually only seek physical health care and not mental health care, and are often underserved because of language barriers and because providers do not understand culturally-specific manifestations of mental health symptoms (Council of National Psychological Associations for the Advancement of Ethnic Minority Interests, 2003). Significant percentages of Native American populations continue to reside on federal reservations and are underserved because they frequently lack of awareness that mental services exist and do not understanding how counseling services work (Council of National Psychological Associations for the Advancement of Ethnic Minority Interests, 2003). They also tend to terminate services after one session because they experience providers as non-responsive and culturally insensitive to native healing traditions and customs (Council of National Psychological Associations for the Advancement of Ethnic Minority Interests, 2003). This is of particular concern because suicide and general death rates are disproportionately high for African-Americans, Latinos, and Native Americans (PBS, 2009). Moffat et al. (2009) report that cultural and ethnic minorities often fail to receive appropriate care at the earliest stages of illness. Knifton et al. (2010) attribute this failure to stigma associated with mental health problems and the manner in which this stigma makes it difficult for cultural minorities to seek professional help (Knifton et al., 2010). This discussion underscores the need for culturally competent mental health services.

My recent experience has been that clinicians are increasingly expected to work competently with cultural minorities. My experience has also been that trainings on diversity topics are more readily available and are often required by public agency personnel departments. Although I find this encouraging, a majority of the trainings I have attended narrowly focus on the presentation of general information about underserved populations and reminding attendees to be respectful and sensitive to differences. Although such information is of course helpful to review, much of it could be considered common knowledge among practicing professionals.

Furthermore, my experience has been that, in cultural competence trainings, there is *never* discussion of the specific realities of doing culturally competent clinical work with vulnerable populations *as a clinician from the dominant, white class.* In particular, I find there is little transparent discussion about techniques that have worked in specific interchanges in specific cases, what has not worked, how positive and negative interchanges may generalize, and a broader discussion and exploration of cross-cultural dynamics in psychotherapy. This is a personal and introspective process that I have found immensely helpful to my own professional development. I have also found that broaching such topics in private dialogue with individual clinicians (of any cultural background) or in cultural competency trainings usually results in avoidant responses.

These aforementioned concerns inspired me to write this text, which includes several cases of vulnerable population clients from my clinical practice. These particular cases strongly contributed to my professional growth and cultural sensitivity, both as a white clinician and as an increasingly self-aware being in a multi-cultural world. I will present these cases along with discussion questions and short assignments at clinically significant points in the cases. I hope this will help my reader get a sense of what it was like to be in the room with the clients under study and then introspect in a way that may inform similar clinical experiences in the future. I will also present my cases alongside clinical theories that helped me formulate treatment and understand what happened in the therapy. I selected theories based on what felt to best capture my therapeutic approach, explain what happened in key interchanges, and hypothesize in a way that provided a helpful guide for future sessions. My hope is that this integration of theory and practice methods will inform the learning of cross-culturally sensitive readers. My broader hope is that this course of study will present a framework for a research-informed operationalization of cultural competency principles.

Writing Assignment: *How can you evaluate your own cultural competence as a clinician and identify when additional training may be necessary? Looking back at your own clinical work history, clients from which ethnic backgrounds have most readily engaged with you and clients from whom ethnic backgrounds have been the most difficult for you to therapeutically engage with? What would you say have been your contributions to the positive outcomes and the negative outcomes?*

Chapter 2

THE PARALLEL PROCESS IMPLICATIONS OF ATTACHMENT THEORY IN CROSS-CULTURAL THERAPY AND CLINICAL SUPERVISION

When I was a first year Master of Social Work intern, I learned that a client's growth as a result of therapy is strongly influenced by the strength of the therapeutic relationship. I also learned that therapeutic growth may be indirectly influenced by the relationship that the clinician has with his or her supervisor.

I learned this when I interned at an inner city public school where I provided therapy to Joey, a severely traumatized teenage African-American foster child. I provided therapy to him under the clinical supervision of Tessa. This supervisory relationship was very challenging for me to navigate, though was also very meaningful to my professional development. In the beginning of each of these relationships, I was very anxious and insecure. As the school year progressed, my relationship with my supervisor seemed to deepen and become more trusting right around the same time that my relationship with Joey seemed to deepen. Of course, causality cannot be inferred and a multitude of relational factors influenced what occurred in the therapy. At the same time, the aforementioned parallel process implications warrant further discussion and exploration.

I will narrate the case of Joey and I, and my clinical supervisor as it occurred in that time period. This will include my ways of thinking about the case during the internship. My hope is that this transparent exploration will help my reader to conceptualize my experience of a profoundly meaningful parallel process. So as to establish a more evidence-based framework for this discussion, I will conceptualize key interchanges in the therapy and supervisory relationship through attachment theory. I have selected this theory because applications of its principles will be shown to generate meaningful hypotheses' about the more clinically significant interchanges in my work with Joey and Tessa.

AN OVERVIEW OF ATTACHMENT THEORY

Infants have innate desires for soothing, touch, and tenderness (Hughes, 2006). When these needs are correctly identified and responded to by primary caregivers, infants feel loved and develop a core sense of trust in others (Bowlby, 1960; 1963, 1969). When infants' needs are misunderstood by primary caregivers and are responded to incorrectly, the resulting relationship rupture provides an opportunity for repair (J. Schore, personal communication, 6/7/2010). Rupture and repair experiences build the neurobiological capacity for affect regulation (Schore, 2003).

When infants' needs are frequently misunderstood and are not repaired, or they are chronically abused or neglected, they go on to develop insecure attachment styles (Ainsworth et al., 1978; Hughes, 2006). The authors note that these styles are informative about their earlier life relational experiences and are invariably self-defeating in future relationships.

Ainsworth et al. (1978) studied the effects of maternal separation and reunion and identified patterns in children's attachment behaviors. Children who are raised by inconsistent, unreliable caregivers are often clingy and hyper sensitive. The authors describe this attachment style as *preoccupied.* Children who are raised by critical and dismissing caregivers are *avoidant* of emotional connection that is nevertheless desired at a deeper level. Children who are raised by chronically abusive and neglectful caregivers develop a *disorganized* style (Main et al., 1986; Cassidy et al., 2008). This latter style is marked by the lack of a coherent attachment strategy, chaotic attempts to forge relationships, and dissociation.

Wallin (2007) contends that the aforementioned model of early life relationships provides a guide for therapy. The author notes that therapy clients frequently present with insecure styles, and need the therapist to facilitate the relational experiences that were lacking in early life. This essentially provides a corrective emotional experience. The preoccupied client needs consistency and soothing, the avoidant client needs to be more actively reached out to and emotionally connected with, and the disorganized client requires stability and grounding. The expectation is that long term, corrective emotional-relational experiences coupled with increased general life stability *may* improve present day relational behavior (Wallin, 2007; Cassidy et al., 2008).

My relationships with Tessa and Joey lasted only one year and were therefore insufficient to redress Joey's longer standing attachment problems or my own, deeper insecurities. Joey's long history of trauma and neglect would require years of therapy and a more stable home life situation than he will be shown to have had. I will nevertheless show that Tessa's supervision provided me with a corrective *professional* experience, which I in turn provided to Joey in the form of rupture and repair experiences.

Writing Assignment: *More highly traumatized, urban inner city clients-of-color are often difficult for European American therapists to engage in therapy. What might attachment theory say about why this is so?*

____

____

____

____

____

____

JOEY, TESSA AND I; THE BEGINNING

When I first began to learn about attachment theory in my master's program, I thought that practicing in accordance with its principles would be easy. I needed *only* to identify my relational style and that of my client, follow the model, and provide my client with a better relational experience than what he or she had typically experienced. Through my experience with Joey and Tessa, I learned that facilitating emotionally attuned therapy is far more challenging.

I met with Joey for approximately 25 sessions at his middle school, where I was in a pseudo-school counseling role. He had been referred to me by his special education teacher because his grades were poor and he struggled with following his teacher's instructions. His math teacher told me that Joey "doesn't listen to anybody." His referent special education teacher told me that his "mind always seems to be elsewhere."

My Arrival

I felt fear, tension, confusion, and despair as I walked into Joey's 8th grade classroom. The school was located in a neighborhood that was plagued with high levels of drugs, crime, poverty, and plight. I had read nightmarish stories of this school and its host community in local newspapers.

When I arrived, I saw dilapidated buildings and met weary teachers. I found resolve by thinking of the kids, and how hard it must be for them to survive in this environment. Rather than trying to imagine, I jolted myself back to reality. Young, inexperienced, and motivated, I was eager to make a difference.

I expected that building a relationship with these children would be difficult. Many of them were referred to me for counseling by school officials who suspected that they had survived severe abuse and neglect at the hands of parents who were *at least* as troubled. These thoughts raced through my mind as I visited the 8th grade classroom for the first time.

As I made my way into a math class, I tried to find comfort in how I might have felt a sense of fear, tension, confusion, and despair that might be ever prevalent in my new internship environment. I observed a group of seven or so girls sitting in the far back row. Some of them were sharing the latest news with each other. Two of them were chattering away on their cell phones, oblivious to the world past the tips of their noses. Two boys teetered back in their chairs and were slumped over apathetically. Most of the students seemed somewhere between a holiday and anarchy: Yelling, cursing, laughing, and almost competing with one another for who could be the most outrageous. Their teacher, biologically 40 or so, seemed to age by the minute. He chased after them, shouting, waving his arms, pleading, screaming, and shaking his head. He was as active as the students, and yet he was invisible to them.

Then I saw a boy who I later learned to be Joey. He was slumped down in his chair and was contemptuous in his posture, yet with a subtle curiosity in his eyes. Something about him told me that it was okay for me to approach. He stared down sorrowfully at his desk as if he wanted to have his thoughts interrupted. I wanted to sit down next to him and ask him, "what's wrong?" I trusted my intuition to try something less intrusive.

I sat down on my heels in front of his desk with my elbows on the edge and my thoughts racing. *Who is this boy? Where is he from? What does he think of me?*

This immediate reaction to Joey might indicate that I was preoccupied. Wallin (2007) noted that preoccupied therapists are overly connected to their own internal processes. This was particularly true when Joey and I began our dialogue. As we made eye contact and made "getting to know you" talk, I grew progressively more anxious.

Nevertheless, Joey surprised me by readily engaging. My own sense of inadequacy was telling me that he would want nothing to do with me. To the contrary, Joey looked up at me with eyes that told me stories of pain and shame. As our eyes locked, he was focused and attentive. I wasn't sure if he was mocking me, testing me, or telling me he needed help in a most intense manner; maybe all three. Nelson (2008) said that a tear communicates *a thousand words*: Though Joey was not teary, making eye contact with him communicated at least that many.

As I tutored him through the math problems on his desk, Joey remained quietly intense for the next half hour. He seemed interested and grateful to be getting some help, though he also seemed distracted. He would sometimes look around the room and stare off into nowhere. When class ended, we barely noticed the other students stampeding out the door. I still didn't yet know what I was doing, but our relationship was beginning away.

A few long minutes after the room was empty, we looked up from Joey's school work. At the same time, we both seemed to notice that we were alone. Somehow, the consciousness shifted. As I introduced myself to Joey as clinical staff, Joey told me that he had a therapist at one point, and that he was sad to recently see this relationship end.

I'm sorry, I said; not to apologize, but to empathize. Speaking spontaneously to Joey in lay terms seemed to help Joey to experience me as a real, supportive other. Looking back, this attuned interchange may have provided an initial comfort zone that Joey and I both needed.

Joey seemed to relax, as evidenced by a softening of his brow and his losing some of its deadness. His eyes widened slightly and he told me that he was ready to *"let it all out"* if I was ready to listen. He locked eyes with me as if daring me to agree. Before I could answer, he breathed in deeply as if bracing himself for the impact of what he was intent on saying. I silently wished I was as ready as Joey said he was.

Joey's Story

As he told me his story, Joey spoke slowly, quietly, and deliberately. His eyes looked large and empty, as if he was devoid of emotion. His voice and facial expression never changed, regardless of what he was talking about. He used a similar tone of voice to describe being abandoned in his early life and to describe turning in his homework late.

He exposed his inner world to me, piece by piece. This included terrifying accounts of inner city drug wars and gang slayings. Taking care of his baby brother Ronnie was all Joey had to keep him distracted. When Joey was busy making sure that she was clothed and fed and played with, he didn't have to feel.

While eight year old Joey was functioning as Ronnie's surrogate parent, his adult family disappeared for days at a time in search of crack cocaine or to avenge the deaths of comrades lost to drug wars. All of this came out in the first five minutes that Joey and I were alone together. Joey had so much to say. Silently, I kept wishing that I could of a word to say to him that might be reassuring, but everything I thought of saying died on my tongue. I was feeling quite overwhelmed by Joey's story.

Discussion Question: *At this point in the case, how would you be feeling if you were Joey's therapist and how might that either help or hinder your therapeutic work with him?*

Looking back on it, my saying nothing was probably the best I could have done. Just being there, being overwhelmed by him, listening, and attempting to metabolize his experiences was the kind of relational experience that Joey needed most from therapy. If this more secure experience was repeated consistently over the course of many years, Joey might learn more secure relational behavior. This hypothesis is consistent with the attachment theories that are described by Wallin (2007). Research supports that attachment disconfirming experiences can help to reconcile early life traumas and object relations (Maltby, 2012).

While I was wished I could find something to say that was reassuring, Joey continued with his story. Throughout his early life, street gangs seemed to be everywhere, killing themselves and innocent civilians. This rendered Joey and Ronnie hostage in their own home, as was familiar to the majority of people in Joey's neighborhood.

Joey described his community as resigned to this desolate state of affairs. Desolation was just the way things were and there was no hope of improvement. I wondered if this was why Joey sat in his English classroom looking so weary. It was as if he was non-verbally saying, "This is as good as it gets and as good as it gets isn't so good." This detachment is consistent with the attachment-disorganized presentation of a child who had been repeatedly traumatized.

In response to Joey's story up to that moment, I felt sad. This emotional response helps to explain why I so badly wanted to say something soothing to him. When I am sad or uncomfortable, I usually respond by getting into action. Meanwhile, we sat in the classroom with a foot of table between us, watching each other closely.

Joey spoke to me with a non-chalance that seemed to come from somewhere between inner strength and despair. It was as if his experiences with violence and poverty were so normal that they were impersonal, yet he was struggling to ward off the traumatic effects. As he spoke about his traumas, his voice didn't change and his posture didn't shift.

Discussion Question: *Consider your personal experiences with African-Americans. What might be some of the cultural implications of Joey's aforementioned survival strategies? How might his survival strategies be misdiagnosed by less culturally competent mental health providers?*

____

____

____

____

____

____

____

A More Thorough History of Joey

I will now present more of the details of Joey's early life history. I am doing so at this point in this paper because I got most of this information at the end of our first session. I did not ask for these details when I first met with Joey (in typical question - answer intake format) because I was concerned that asking Joey for sensitive information might make him uncomfortable. Therefore, I decided to let him decide what we would discuss. In a sense, this was good mothering.

Joey was a pre-teen age African American male from the South Bronx in New York. He was removed from his parents' custody when he was five and was in several foster care placements until age 10. It was then that he secured a permanent placement.

I was unaware of the details of his multiple foster care placements, including lengths of stay and reasons for transfer. I hypothesize that he may have had conduct problems, which would be consistent with his conduct problems at school and is somewhat predicted by chronic early life neglect (Hughes, 2006).

Conceptualizing Joey through Attachment Theory

Joey's strong attempts to connect with me, early life neglect, detached-dissociated presentation, observed difficulty concentrating, problems in school, and labile affect suggest a preoccupied-disorganized style. This would be consistent with his preoccupied presentation when we first met. Joey made strong attempts to engage with me though detached from the content of his story. This may have been his way of attempting to facilitate relational proximity by being a "good therapy client" and disclosing readily, though also protecting himself from painful affects. According to Wallin (2007), this would suggest that Joey had particular attachment needs for reliable, soothing, and consistent caregiving. In therapy, these needs can be met through attunement to nonverbal cues, as well as rupture and repair experiences. These experiences would help to facilitate affect regulation. This is an example of how attachment theory can be used to hypothesize about a client's early life and what was missing from those experiences, which then informs the therapist about what the client needs from the therapeutic relationship.

My Beginning with Tessa

When I first met Tessa, I remember feeling slightly pushed back by her smaller stature and a strong demeanor that was not unlike my mothers'. Both were quietly alert and stoic, though with a slightly skeptical psychology that made me insecure and eager to win approval. When I first met Tessa, I appreciated her energy and outwardly warm demeanor, though I also intuitively sensed something ominous about her that made me feel the need to remain on guard.

I usually began supervision by presenting detailed notes of what occurred in my sessions. I often recounted the more favorable outcomes of my various attempts to help my child clients get well. I beamed at Tessa's approvals and fearfully anticipated her rejection. She always seemed to give me the approval I wanted, and I responded with outward gratification. I also harbored a deeper underlying mistrust and was waiting for a harder truth to be revealed. Something like this was a pattern I remember well in my early life.

The Middle of the School Year

Throughout the first half of the school year, Joey described his present day life as if he was fighting to survive in the present, as he had in the past. When he told me about his memories of gang wars and drug deals, he often used the present tense. This may suggest that his neurological capacities were severely disrupted by trauma.

Joey presented as battle weary. His affect was flat, his posture was slumped, and he tended to rapidly and anxiously shift from one topic to the next. It was hard for me to see him suffer so immensely and to be so frantic, afraid, and desperate.

As noted previously, I often wished I had something reassuring to say. Though I was unaware at the time, Joey probably had people in his life who tried to say things that were reassuring in effort to make him feel better. My role was to let him talk and track his feelings, to be reliable and emotionally available, to share laughs and smiles with him, and to otherwise connect with him in right-brained ways that would help him regulate his affect and parallel a secure mother-infant dyad. This conceptualization is supported by an attachment theory of therapy (Schore et al. 2008; Wallin, 2007).

Discussion Question: *Consider your clinical experiences with African-American clients. Do your instincts usually lead you, in the early stages of treatment, to ask a significant number of informational – intake questions or to hesitate to ask what might be considered a good number of informational questions? How might your natural instincts be helpful and/or harmful to the clinical work?*

In sessions 10 through 15, I began to more clearly witness Joey's lack of regulatory capacities. He would sometimes talk about one trauma after another in rapid succession. He would talk about his brother who he had lost contact with, then mention shootings that happened in his old neighborhood, and then discuss conflicts he was having with his foster parents. His eyes would grow wider, he would break the intense eye contact we normally maintained, and his muscles would tense. His voice would subtly quicken. At the same time, I remember my own heart beat speeding up and feeling a suddenly frantic energy. Sensing that Joey was overwhelmed (and maybe because I was too), I would often step in and be more therapeutically active in those moments. An example of what I would say is as follows:

"That all must have been so hard for you, and it must have seemed like it would never end. You were hurt over and over again and so it makes sense that you find yourself going over these thoughts and feelings again and again almost as if these events are happening over and over again. When people are hurt very badly, they often re-live those terrifying events. Your feelings are normal given what you have been through. As heavy of an experience as all of this has been for you, there is much to be hopeful for. I have seen a strength and toughness in you that not only helped you protect yourself and your brother through the danger you faced, but also to walk through these doors so as to face and talk about your fears. We will untangle them one by one, make some sense out of what we can, help you develop a plan for how to deal with this stuff when it comes up, and little by little, you might just start feeling better." When I would say such things, Joey would stare at me hard. He looked like he was deep in thought. Then he would say nothing for a few long seconds, and change the subject.

I was never certain what he was thinking about, though I had the sense that he got the gist of what I was trying to tell him. It could have been that my intervention was too long and complicated for him to follow and influenced by my own need to regulate myself by becoming more active. It was also important for Joey to experience something like responsive caregiving. As a more experienced clinician, I would probably allow more space for Joey to explore his experiences, track his feelings, and decrease verbosity. As a first year MSW intern, I was giving Joey the best mothering I was capable of. This is supported by Hughes (2006) to be the ultimate need of severely traumatized, attachment-disorganized children.

Assessment of What Was Happening in Therapy

When I was supportive of Joey, he would often look at me like he wanted to believe me. His wary eyes seemed to scan me for truth. *Do you really mean it?* He seemed to be thinking.

In a way, I shared this non-verbal skepticism with him. I didn't distrust my positive regard, but I sometimes doubted whether I could help him. I experienced a lot of insecurities in my work with Joey. I now attribute these insecurities, in part, to my being a less experienced clinician. Additionally, Joey's emotional pain and the extent of his trauma history sometimes lead me to feel overwhelmed and a sense of despair. Despite our best efforts to achieve regulation as individuals, our relationship was demonstrating one of the primary principles of attachment: When emotions overwhelm neurobiological capacities, a stable and reliable caregiving figure is needed.

Discussion Question: *How might Joey's weariness be culturally appropriate?*

____

____

____

The Middle of the Road with Tessa

Halfway through the school year, more of my blunders as an intern were beginning to leak out into supervision. I remained eager to win Tessa's approval, which I sometimes pursued through devising complex theoretical conceptualizations of what was happening in the lives of my child clients. I cannot remember any one in particular, though I do remember overthinking what was occurring in my sessions with Joey and being scolded in response. I outwardly attempted to maintain my composure, though tended to shut down and detach emotionally in a way that rendered me only so emotionally present in supervision. As Tessa and I grew further apart, my insecurities about my competence grew and I considered quitting. Meanwhile, it felt as if I was on my own with Joey.

Session 16

Nearly three-quarters of the way through the school year, Joey told me about a time that he walked to a corner store. In his words, "the past came back to haunt me." On his walk, he saw a house that reminded him of a house that his aunt had taken him to when he was eight years old. She had taken him there because she wanted to buy crack, but did not want to leave him alone and *in danger*. In this crack house, the floor was littered with trash mounds and the floor and living room sofa were damp. On that sofa, and on top of each other, were two naked, heavy set lesbians, lost in pleasure and undeterred by Joey's eight year old presence mere feet away from them. Joey stood there, awkwardly looking away. He seemed to feel humiliated and confused.

Five years later, Joey walked was walking to the corner store with me and passed a house that *looked like* that same crack house that was just described. Each house was painted white, the paint was chipped, and there were broken toys in the yard. But to Joey, they were the same.

As Joey told me about this experience, his speech quickened and he began to breathe more heavily. He told me that, when he was eight and in the crack house, he felt like a prisoner in that living room. He wished that he could turn invisible and leave his humiliation behind. In session, he looked off to the horizon with intense fear, wide eyes, on setting tears, and clamming skin. He cried out loudly (about his intrusive memories): *"Why can't they just stop!?!?!"*

Joey was uncharacteristically emotional at this point. We were suddenly only inches apart, but we could not look at each other. We both sat there, overwhelmed, and breathing hard. I remember Joey looking really scared and confused, but I also remember him leaning towards me as if trying to draw strength. This would be consistent with the attachment theory of early life proximity seeking that Wallin (2007) applies to therapeutic relational dynamics.

In session 16, Joey's terror and overwhelm were powerful and frightening. I too struggled to stay present, but I intuitively knew that I needed to stay out of Joey's way and let him feel his feelings. Looking back on it, I was *"with Joey"* moment to moment. I was frantic and overwhelmed for he was frantic and overwhelmed.

I hoped that my effort to hold the space and contain myself was enough for both of us. My reaction was particularly strong because Joey had often seemed so distant and detached. In previous sessions, his emotional intensity was more subtle. He would make intense eye contact, display signs of muscular tension, and speak in ominous tones. But Joey's speech and affect were usually impoverished.

As Joey told me about his experience of walking to the corner store, he seemed to become re-traumatized. I may have been feeling some of the feelings that he had previously kept at bay. This description is consistent with the theory of projection, a defensive structure that is expected of one with a traumatic early life history. As I struggled internally, Joey looked fragile and split open. I was also in survival mode and mentally searched myself for how to handle this experience. I hated not knowing "what to do" and remember feeling intensely panic-stricken. In those long moments, our self-soothing skills were unable to help us. For Joey, self-soothing usually meant detaching. For me, self-soothing usually meant becoming very active. But this time was different. This time, we sat there and felt.

Joey cried heavy tears, breathed hard, and said very little. Searching for an answer, I suggested that we take a walk around the block to help him (and possibly myself) calm down. I remember feeling as afraid as he looked. I watched him closely: His far off stare, and his stumbling and awkward steps. He looked like he was in another world. But I felt like I was there with him. As we took our walk, we were emotional, raw, and saying nothing because there might not be anything that needed to be said.

We had both calmed down by the time we returned to the school campus 5 minutes later. By the end of our walk, Joey was speaking in a normal tone of voice and was able to make socially appropriate eye contact. I also felt like I was getting back on the ground again.

He reported that he felt well enough to go back to class. We exchanged grim smiles and waved goodbye. I wanted to smile in relief, but I was still shaken up. The suddenness of it all had gotten to me.

Immediately thereafter, Joey began to ask for extra weekly therapy sessions. Looking back on it, I take this as a sign that he was beginning to trust me. This last interchange and

Joey's positive response is consistent with the attachment theory of affect regulation (Schore et al., 2008).

A psychodynamic therapist might object to my response to Joey's projective process on the premise that I was defensively responding to counter transference. Looking back on this session, my intense overwhelm and more instinctive response was typical of a lesser experienced intern. Nevertheless, Joey's regulated response might suggest that the ends justified the means. Neurobiological research on trauma also supports that recovery is facilitated when therapy helps clients give a full account of trauma and work through it therapeutically (Van der kolk, 2012). It was important for Joey to revisit his trauma, feel related feelings, and then regulate.

My Experience with Joey Seeping Into Supervision with Tessa

I remember feeling more self-assured with the results of session 16. I was also beginning to feel mightily fed up with what felt like a multitude of unproductive supervisory sessions with Tessa. In the beginning of the year I was certain that her criticisms were unquestionably founded. By the middle of the year, I became more aware of my incremental successes and that my resentment about Tessa interfered with my ability to use her as a resource for my professional development. I knew she was knowledgeable about psychotherapy with young teen African-American populations and resolved myself to try to work things out with her directly. This more assertive problem solving strategy has helped me develop secondary relationships that somewhat compensate for my own earlier life ruptures. Although I remain sensitive to rejection and dislike, I have learned through experience to see past my own hyper activated feelings and to work towards secure relational experiences. In turn, this helps me to feel more secure about myself.

With such experiences intuitively in mind, I nervously called Tessa. I was completely unsure of what to expect, though I was certain that our relationship had to change, for my sake and for the sake of Joey's therapy. I breathed deeply as she answered the phone with my hand slightly shaking. I asked her if she would be gentler with me in supervision sessions. Much to my relief, Tessa stammered, paused, and agreed. I was even more pleased to see that she consistently granted what I asked for. She never apologized for telling me various harder truths, but she also tended to interact with me without the anger that struck chords that were painfully familiar to my early life experiences.

What Happened Next

At the end of session 16, Joey and I were both more regulated and I felt like I was "out of the woods." However, I learned that, once a client safely works through a trauma in session, he or she may want to talk about other traumas. This may occur because trust has been built and the client now feels safe enough to explore further. This also parallels the attachment theory of development: When an infant trusts the primary caregiver, he or she will feel more confident about exploring the surrounding environment (Ainsworth et al., 1978). Trust makes this exploration possible because the infant has learned that the primary caregiver can be called upon in times of crisis (Hughes, 2006). If exploring the unknown ever becomes frightening or otherwise too much to handle, the secure infant need only engage in an attachment behavior (such as crying). In turn, the caregiver will provide proximity which will help to resolve the fear and help the infant regulate his or her affect (Nelson, 2008). This is not meant to say that Joey developed internal security. Rather, he had an experience with me that is consistent with the rupture and repair experiences that build affect regulatory capacities (Schore et al., 2008). In Joey's case, he undertook a more secure exploration of his present-day experiences, as opposed to becoming overwhelmed by traumatic memories.

Soon after session 16, Joey told me and his special education teacher that he had been physically abused by his foster father. Joey told me that his pervasively poor grades had become a source of tension and ongoing debate at home. One night, the usual argument over academics escalated. Joey became loud and defiant when his foster father demanded that he do his homework. His foster father retaliated by beating him across the back with a belt. As a mandated reporter of child abuse, I informed Joey that I had to make a CPS report.

Discussion Question: Given what you know at this point, if you were the CPS worker assigned to Joey's families' case, what would be your case plan? What would be the pros and cons of your plan? Consider relevant cultural factors.

The system takes abuse very seriously when the survivor is already in the foster care system. Therefore, I anticipated that a follow up investigation must have occurred, though I do not know for certain what happened as a result of my report.

It has been my professional experience in working with African-American foster youth that they tend to be well aware that clinical staff will report abuse to the authorities. Thus, I expect that Joey may have known what I and his special education teacher were likely to do when he informed us of the abuse. Furthermore, it is possible that he told me about what his foster father did to him because he trusted me to take action.

Despite the physical abuse, Joey's special education teacher and I were hopeful that Joey would not be removed from his current placement. Instead, we hoped that the family would receive services that would help make this placement work. Joey reported that his foster father planned to adopt him, had physically abused him just that one time, and they usually had a good relationship. Additionally, Joey's age and behavioral problems made it unlikely that he would be adopted by another family. If he were removed from his foster father's home, he might have spent the remainder of his youth in group homes. This would also be another traumatic loss.

More about Joey's History of Separation

As the school year progressed, Joey told me more of the details of his past. After being permanently separated from his biological family, he was moved from temporary foster home to temporary foster home throughout his early life. His brother had similarly unstable foster placements due to behavioral problems, which eventually lead them to lose touch. Joey reported having no idea where he was and quickly changed the subject.

He did report a particularly meaningful relationship with a foster mother in Florida. He described her as kind, though also strong and perceptive. She was quick to scold him for bad behavior, though also explained clearly what was expected of him at home and at school. They often went to movies together and learned to relate as biological mother and son. The foster mother's equal mix of tough and love lead Joey to love and respect her dearly.

After a year of living happily with her, Joey's social worker informed him that he was scheduled for an out-of-state interview for adoption with his current foster-adoptive family. The social worker and his beloved foster mother attempted to explain to Joey why this was a good move for him. They explained that the move was not indicative that his foster mother did not love him, or that he had done anything wrong. Nevertheless, Joey talked to me about this separation as if it were a result of his failure to behave properly. He asked himself questions he couldn't answer about why he didn't get better grades or remember to do his chores. Hughes (2006) noted that children who experience trauma and attachment problems often blame themselves for what happened and develop a core sense of pervasive shame. Multiple primary relational separations provide near-causal explanations for Joey's disorganized-preoccupied relational behavior. The ongoing story of Joey's life was that anyone special who came into his life would eventually leave him.

Discussion Question: *Knowing what you <u>now</u> know about Joey, revisit the previous hypothetical of your being Joey's families' assigned CPS worker. Would you now propose any changes to your original CPS case plan? Please explain why or why not.*

____

____

____

____

____

____

____

As Joey told me about these experiences, I felt a similar sense of shame. Joey felt like he failed to protect his brother and to behave good enough to maintain his foster placement. I felt like a failure for not being able to protect Joey from his feelings and from his memories. Again, I felt like I was supposed to *do something*. As discussed previously, this could be attributed to my lack of clinical experience. This may also suggest that I was in a pre-occupied state: In key interchanges with Joey, I was overwhelmed and panic-stricken. Wallin

(2007) noted that a therapist may be preoccupied if he or she is unable to do more than empathize. I often struggled to maintain my composure, though I sought to remain as calm as possible so that Joey would not see that he was causing me distress. Joey needed a strong, emotionally available caregiver to help him hold himself together. By this point, so did I.

Bringing My Relationship with Joey into My Relationship with Tessa

A few sessions after Joey's fairly productive trauma processing, my initial glow was wearing off. I became more aware of Joey's ongoing behavior problems in class, poor grades, and quarrels with his peers. I was having a particularly hard time with my impression that *Joey seemed to be suffering more* rather than feeling better. It is possible that he might incrementally be "feeling worse" because he was beginning to work through experiences that had to be processed in order to facilitate healing. As a younger, less experienced intern, I was disappointed to not see quick, easily observable behavior changes.

I went to Tessa, feeling anxious and confused. I was talking rapidly and fidgeting. She looked at me with calm and reassuring eyes, sitting back in her chair, and never interrupting me. She was supportive and nurturing in her own way, as I was to Joey. I asked her fearfully if I was *"doing the right thing,"* having run out of my own ideas of how to "keep things under control" and sharing (with her) my feelings of inadequacy. I spoke in a rapid and shaky voice, making uncharacteristically little eye contact, mixing a lot of "ums" into what I was trying to say, and probably only making coherent sense for about 10 of the 20 minutes that I was talking to her. I do remember that most of what I had to say pertained to my being afraid of failure: In my work with Joey, and in my internship on the whole.

She sat back, nodding her head slightly, taking me in, and normalizing some of my feelings. She neither reinforced nor tried to assuage my insecurities. That experience was relieving, particularly because I was not chastised for being incompetent (as I learned to expect in both my experiences with her and in my own early life).

As I calmed in supervision, Tessa gently pushed me in the direction of exploring my reactions and feelings which related to my work with Joey. That's when we identified that my feelings of internal chaos, anxiety, fear, failure and the like may have been what Joey was feeling. He sometimes had difficulty expressing his feelings and lacked affect regulatory capacities. My supervisor suggested that Joey's feelings were basically flooding out of him and that I might be taking them in and feeling them with him. Rather than being indicative of failure, Tessa's position was that we might ultimately be doing "good therapy." This realization helped me to feel like I was back on the ground again, paralleling session 16 of therapy with Joey and disconfirming my own pattern attachment experiences. Maybe this is why I remember this supervision session so well. Ultimately, Tessa provided a parallel of a secure base from which my exploration occurred. It was here that I learned how to really use supervision. Interestingly, my exploration, return to safety, and more confident exploration in the future parallels Ainsworth et al.'s (1978) theories of secure separation-reunion behavior. The authors found that secure infants explore their environment and return to their caregivers when afraid. When they are securely responded to, they develop a trust in the caregiver. This sense of trust translates into a willingness to explore more readily on the premise that they can always return to safety as needed.

I thought more deeply about this sequence of events later that week and speculated that not asking Tessa for her help (due to my own insecurities) was interfering with my professional development, as well as Joey's progress in therapy. As I wanted to help Joey heal and I also wanted to grow as a clinician, I made a commitment to myself to be more forthcoming with Tessa about what was happening in therapy sessions. This parallels Bowlby's (1969) contention that receiving needed support and proximity from trusted others allows for a secure sense of self-confidence in one's ability to move into greater levels of independence.

Termination: Saying Goodbye

It was now the end of the school year, which meant that Joey and I would be saying goodbye to each other. He asked if we could stay in touch via me being his mentor, and I was thrilled at that possibility. I remembered that my supervisor had told me that she kept in limited contact with a couple of inner city foster children who she had worked with a long time ago. In turn, I was hopeful that I could such an ongoing contact with Joey.

Discussion Question: *Given Joey's history, why would it be therapeutic to have ongoing contact with him and why might it be therapeutic to more formally terminate? At this point, what would you recommend and why?*

____

____

____

____

____

____

____

It was hard for me to hear Tessa tell me, *"no, you need to learn how to go through termination with your clients, and Joey needs to learn how to have healthy goodbyes."* I protested on the basis that Joey had many severed attachment relationships: His brother, his beloved foster mother, his parents, his ex-therapist, and now me too?

My supervisor agreed that Joey needed long term bonding experiences, but that primary male bonding needed to happen with his adoptive-foster father. As I could see her point, I conceded, but with a heaviness in my heart. I knew I would miss Joey greatly.

In addition to my loss of Joey, I was also grieving my loss of Tessa. Saying goodbye to her was almost equally painful. Looking back on it, when I tried to convince her to let me stay in touch with Joey, this may have been my way of protesting *both losses.*

After this last supervision session, I met with Joey and reluctantly informed him that we would not be staying in contact. I acknowledged that he needed to bond with his foster father and have a healthy, non-traumatic experience of saying goodbye. Later that day, I saw him sitting down on the steps outside of the school, looking as sad as I felt.

This termination was therapeutic for Joey given that it provided him with the experience of a goodbye that didn't involve a funeral or an abrupt separation. Additionally, he had an opportunity to *feel* rather than detach and act out later. His history of separation suggests that he would have a hard time with our termination, regardless of my best efforts.

However, I made it worse by not talking to him about termination until the end of the year because of my own fears of loss and separation. Tessa rightly chastised me for this. So as to address this issue, I told Joey that I should have brought up termination with him sooner and that I didn't because saying goodbye to him would be painful for me. He looked away and nodded in resignation: A nod that told me that he knew what I meant and could relate. Our behavior during the termination phase of Joey's therapy may be further evidence that we were both preoccupied. Alternatively, our mutual sadness also could have been the movingly human result of two young men bonding, connecting, and having to say goodbye.

Conclusion: What Did I Learn?

In addition to learning how to say goodbye to clients, I learned something about what it was like to be a client and to have what almost felt like a corrective attachment experience with Tessa. In both therapy with Joey and supervision with Tessa, rupture and repair experiences helped to facilitate regulation and *intermittently* more secure relational behavior. As a result of being in relationships with both of them, I learned more about how to trust and be trusted in a professional context. I also learned the intrinsic value of using proximity to provide soothing, as well as how to use a caregiver (my supervisor) to trust, explore, and say goodbye to a relationship I hated to let go of. It was this experience that helped me work more effectively with Joey. I grew not only as a practitioner, but as a person.

Chapter 3

BLACK, WHITE, AND SHADES OF GRAY: DOING PSYCHOTHERAPY WITH AFRICAN AMERICANS AS A EUROPEAN AMERICAN THERAPIST*

INTRODUCTION

I am a white male who was raised in a predominantly African American community. Reflections on my experiences in this community inspired my longstanding interest in cross-cultural issues in psychotherapy. When I decided to write this chapter, I searched for a theory that could help me formulate my discussion. I reflected on my aforementioned personal experiences and remembered that interpersonal traumas (such as child abuse and spousal abuse) happened frequently. I also considered that a majority of people in my old neighborhood were near always healing from pre-existing traumatic wounds or responding to new and imminent threats. These points led me to conclude that trauma theory was the most appropriate theoretical base for my discussion.

In the following chapter, I will present a general theory of trauma and then briefly discuss child abuse and spousal abuse. I am selecting these particular traumas because they are somewhat common in African American communities (Parham et al., 1999). I will also show that the effects of chronic child and spousal abuse parallel how African-Americans (and lower income, urban African Americans in particular) are affected by white racism. I will then present a black psychological theory of white racism and its historically traumatic effects on African American identify development. These effects will be shown to manifest in barriers to therapeutic engagement when African Americans are paired with white therapists. Next, I will present a few cases from my practice in which intuitively building on African Americans historically-rooted survival strategies lead to increased engagement and positive outcomes. Interestingly, this suggests a culturally specific theory of trauma recovery.

---

* A version of this chapter was also published in *The Journal of Theory Construction & Testing*, Volume 16 Number 1, Published by Tucker Publications. It has been expanded in an effort to encourage wider dissemination of research on the subject.

Discussion Question: *What specific challenges have you faced in therapeutically engaging African American clients? Might your challenges have broader cultural implications? If so, please discuss.*

____

____

____

____

____

____

____

TRAUMA

Kimmerling et al. (2002) noted that an event is considered a trauma when the event threatens the survivor with serious bodily injury or death, or a perceived threat of that magnitude. A traumatic threat is too much for the mind and body to handle, which results in overwhelming terror, confusion, and helplessness (Lieberman et al., 2008). Neurobiologically, this occurs because the sheer magnitude of trauma overwhelms the affect regulatory system, which would normally allow people to face a majority of everyday stimuli, interpret the stimuli, and then respond in ways that maintain emotional regulation.

When a traumatic threat overwhelms the regulatory system, the mind and body go into a state of panic and that manifests in the survival-oriented "flight or fight" state (Lieberman et al., 2008). In this state, survivors are hyper vigilant to subtle changes in their surrounding environments, including fast movements, loud speech or noises, or changes in their physical proximity to others. Hyper vigilance readies traumatized individuals to take quick and decisive action in order to protect themselves.

High levels of arousal can also lead to health problems (Lieberman et al., 2008). Maintaining high levels of arousal requires significant physiological energy, which the mind and body supply by re-routing energy that would normally go into other vitally necessary systems. Thus, maintaining high levels of arousal deprives other mind and body systems needed energy, which eventually leads to impairments.

Kimmerling et al. (20002) noted that the posttraumatic state of hyper arousal/hyper vigilance is the core physiological symptom of posttraumatic stress disorder/PTSD. I will first talk about what posttraumatic pathology looks like in a more narrative sense and then describe the primary symptoms. Posttraumatic symptoms are more likely to manifest and in increasingly severe forms when the survivor is traumatized: repeatedly, by another person, and particularly when the survivor and perpetrator are intimately acquainted. When the violation of trust is more severe and/or chronic, the symptomology tends to be more severe.

Hughes (2006), Briere et al., (2006), Lieberman et al. (2008), Herman (1996), and Kimmerling et al. (2002) all describe survivors of chronic interpersonal trauma as tending to have perpetrators who they are intimately acquainted with. The subgroups of chronic trauma survivors that were discussed the most often in the aforementioned sources were children who are chronically physically abused by a parent and women who are chronically victimized by their intimate partners.

Chronically abused women and chronically physically abused children are emotionally predisposed to seek proximity with their most idealized others, *who are also most likely to traumatize them again* (Lieberman et al., 2008; Kimmerling et al. 2002). Lieberman et al. (2008) described survivors of chronic interpersonal trauma (who necessarily remain in close proximity to their abusers) as being in an *emotional dilemma.* This paradox leads chronic survivors to experience high levels of confusion and anxiety, particularly when they are in close proximity to their perpetrators. In effort to survive, chronically abused women or children may seek the abuser's approval, attempt to bargain for safety, or *act out in ways that provoke negative responses.* I will now discuss what this last symptom looks like for chronically abused children and chronically abused women.

Hughes (2006) described chronically abused children as tending to blame themselves for their abuse. This deeper sense of shame may lead them to provoke strongly negative responses from otherwise caring others. The underlying motivation is to reinforce that other people cannot be trusted and that the abused child can only count on him or herself. This tends to be the chronically abused children's core survival strategy, though invariably destroys relationships. This pattern negative outcome reinforces abused children's core senses of *pervasive shame and unloveability*; which Herman (1996) noted to be a typical affective state of trauma survivors in general.

Lieberman et al. (2008) described abused children's chronic acting out behaviors as their best efforts to protect their abusive parent's necessarily exalted positions. Abusive parents tend to have the most power in the family; particularly because the non-abusive parent may also be abused by the abusive parent or is polarized in fear. Thus, the abusive parent is the families' only reliable source of security, direction, and identity. Therefore, if the abuser was seen as *the problem,* the abused child would feel an unbearable sense of despair to which abuse is at least expected and familiar (Lieberman et al., 2008; McNally, 2007). Abused children may cope with their abuse by acting out or dissociating completely from traumatic memories; which may be necessary for survival, though is also a symptom of PTSD and increases vulnerability to further abuse (Lieberman et al., 2008; McNally, 2007).

Similarly, Kimmerling et al. (2002) describes chronically physically abused women as often provoking abusive behavior in their intimate-partner relationships or at least getting into situations where they are likely to be physically abused again. Chronically physically abused women may see themselves as deserving of their abuse. They may also misinterpret abuse as a sign of love, devotion, and a deeper sense of connection and interest. This way of thinking is a survival strategy (like dissociation in children) because it keeps *the abusive nature of the abuse* out of consciousness. This is often necessary because survivors of chronically physically abused women tend to be emotionally and financially dependent on their abusers. Thus, keeping the abuse out of consciousness protects the relationship that is necessary for *and yet also threatens* survival. This discussion shows that both chronically physically abused children and chronically physically abused women (e.g. the two most common subtypes of chronic interpersonal trauma survivors) necessarily develop survival strategies that may *re-create* their victimhood, the other core symptom of posttraumatic stress disorder (PTSD).

PTSD has long been recognized as an anxiety disorder that is neurophysiologically expressed through hyper vigilance to stimuli that is in some way reminiscent of the survivors' trauma and therefore assessed to be threatening (Kimmerling et al, 2002). A trauma survivor with PTSD will usually respond to traumatic stimulus by trying to re-create the trauma (including by having nightmares), avoiding it, emotionally detaching, behaving aggressively, emotionally numbing, or becoming highly anxious and /or agitated (Briere et al., 2006; Lieberman et al., 2008). Trauma survivors who have developed PTSD have learned through experience to expect danger at any time and without warning. Thus, they learn to survive by responding strongly and pre-emptively to potential threats.

Chronic trauma may damage the neurobiological processes that would normally allow relatively more physiologically stable people to more accurately interpret stimuli as either safe or threatening and respond appropriately. Survivors may erroneously interpret subtle changes in their surrounding environments as threatening, respond strongly and pre-emptively, and then remain highly aroused, reactive, and agitated. This can create significant problems in chronic trauma survivors' romantic relationships, family, and workplace (Lieberman et al., 2008; Hughes, 2006). Herman (1996) noted that posttraumatic pathology invariably leads to relational failures, which may lead trauma survivors to isolate and become vulnerable to depression and substance abuse problems.

Now that I have discussed posttraumatic symptomology, I will present a theory of trauma recovery. The key stages in the naturally occurring, bodily process of recovery will be shown to form the principular basis of trauma treatment. Herman (1996) described the trauma recovery process as different for every individual, though also containing pattern elements.

Herman (1996) described trauma recovery as occurring in stages that parallel the stages in Maslow's hierarchy of needs. First, the trauma survivor needs to get out of physical danger and into an environment that is safe and stable. Once physical safety has been re-established, the survivors' emotional needs can be addressed. The survivors' highest priority emotional need is to re-build the core of trust and safety that was built in early life (assuming normal development) and shattered by the trauma. Trust and emotional safety need to be re-built through the reassurance, patience, support, and nurturing of caring others (including the therapist). Lieberman et al. (2008) noted that re-establishing emotional safety facilitates mind and body regulation, which re-routes physiological energy from hyper arousal maintenance to bodily systems. Thus, meeting trauma survivor's emotional needs helps to facilitate physiological recovery.

Herman (1996) noted that chronic trauma survivors' often present in a state of irritability, anxiety, panic, and emotional volatility and reactivity. This can make it extremely difficult for supportive and sensitive others to remain patient and soothing. This is why Herman (1996) emphasized that trauma survivors need to re-connect with their families. It also supports Hughes' (2006) recommendation that trauma survivors work with therapists who will not overly personalize their volatility that naturally follows a traumatic experience.

When I have worked with clients who have recently survived traumas, I have often found it helpful to host family sessions. With all family members present, I have sometimes provided the family members with psycho education (in front of the trauma survivor) about the effects of trauma and what emotional states the survivor is likely to be in. I have then recommended that the loved ones care for the survivor as someone who is physically sick. This speaks to Herman's (1996) recommendation that trauma survivors and their supportive others receive trauma debriefing. My experience has been that this initial intervention can be very effective when the survivor has a supportive family.

Absent debriefing, I have observed that trauma survivors' intense and chaotic emotional states tend to frustrate and overwhelm their usually supportive others. This may result in pervasive relational conflict, which survivors often blame themselves for as described previously. Herman (1996) cautions that self-blaming trauma survivors may then isolate from the social support they need in order to recover.

When a survivors' physical and emotional needs have been addressed, they need to mentally *make sense* of their traumas (Briere et al., 2006). This can occur by connecting a traumatic experience to the similarly traumatic experiences of like-others (Briere et al., 2006; Lieberman et al., 2008). Herman (1996) recommends that this cognitive phase of treatment occur in group therapy. In this phase, therapists help survivors re-examine erroneous self-blame and look more deeply at cognitive distortions that invariably re-create victimhood. The goal in this stage of treatment is to construct a more empathic and realistic narrative.

When trauma survivors have re-established safety and security, and have reconstructed their narrative of their trauma, they will be better able to move on with their lives (Kimmerling et al., 2002). Otherwise, they would remain *mentally and emotionally trapped in their traumatic pasts;* which is another way to conceptualize PTSD (Kimmerling et al., 2002; Briere et al., 2006).

Discussion Question: *How might the process of trauma recovery be unique for African Americans?*

____

____

____

____

I will now present theories of trauma that are more specifically-focused on African-Americans. These *Afro-centric* theories will be shown to take the trauma theories a step further in a culturally-focused direction by naming *white racism* as a trauma. I will then demonstrate that its effects can parallel how women and children are affected by chronic physical abuse. Then, I will present a black psychology theory of how African-Americans can begin to heal and move on with their lives. The integration of these theories will be shown to form the basis for an Afro-centric theory of trauma recovery.

The trauma-focused sources that were cited in my previous section often acknowledged that lower income, urban African-American women and children are at increased risk for being chronically physically abused, though these sources mentioned very little about how white racism contributes to their at-risk status. When the trauma-focused sources did mention the effects of racism /discrimination on African-Americans, the sources described racism as if it has an *emotionally injurious effect*. Parham et al. (1999) goes a step further by defining white racism as a *traumatic threat* to African-Americans (and particularly lower-income, urban African-Americans). Lum (2003) noted white racism threatens their *collective* survival in the present, as it has throughout history. The author noted that white racism inhibits African Americans access to vitally necessary resources. Parham et al. (1999) noted that white racism can negatively skew African American development, which may interfere with employability and lead to depression and posttraumatic hyper sensitivities. On this basis, white racism can be argued to meet criteria for a trauma and create risk for the development of posttraumatic symptoms.

The aforementioned conceptualization of African Americans as traumatically influenced by white racism coincides with the core principles of *Black Psychology* (Parham et al, 1999). This discipline which operates from the premise that African Americans have a completely different worldview and value system than the white mainstream majority (Parham et al., 1999). Afro-centric values include a deeper sense of spirituality and interdependence with nature and other living things, and more highly value emotional expression, direct communication, and expressing one's true emotional self through dance, music, and other creative arts (Parham et al., 1999; Robinson, 1995; Lum, 2003). Parham et al. (1999) emphasized that African Americans need to celebrate the positive attributes of their blackness, which will help them preserve a more positive view of themselves as black people.

The latter authors stress that positivity about one's blackness is vitally necessary to African-Americans' development because their black selves are constantly attacked by the pervasive influence of white racism; which sends subtle and yet powerfully negative messages about blackness in the mainstream media and in everyday social interactions. Negative messages include associating the color black with evil or badness, stereotypes of African Americans as aggressive and lazy, and the systematic promotion of the white mainstreams' values for individualism and competition, rational thought, suppression of emotions, and indirect communication as superior to Afro-centric values and worldview (Parham et al., 1999; Robinson, 1995; Young, 2004). Other examples of this racist influence include the way in which African Americans (and particularly lower income, urban African Americans) are often assumed to be shoplifters rather than customers when entering retail stores (Parham et al., 1999). Discrimination continues to occur in employment, education, and health care, regardless of individualized characteristics such as education and socio-economic status (Waites, 2004; Parham et al., 1999; Robinson, 1995; Sue, 2000; Lum, 2003). Parham et al. (1999) describes the totality of these circumstances as unique to African Americans, which leads them to band together and identify collectively *as black people* a showing of sensitivity to one another's traumatic suffering. This parallels the trauma-oriented theory of how it can be healing for survivors to connect their traumatic experiences to the similarly traumatic experiences of like-others.

At the same time, Wilson (2009) cautioned that, when African-Americans overly identify with an oppressed-identity, they can become hyper sensitive to racism and then overreact in ways that create additional problems. This last point parallels the trauma theory of recreation that has been shown to capture the pathology of chronically physically abused women and children. In both instances, heightened sensitivities may be self-protective, though often self-destructive. As an example of what this posttraumatic hyper sensitivity may look like for African Americans, Alleyne (2004a) and Alleyne (2004b) studied African-Americans experiences in the workplace and found that African Americans who had discriminatory experiences in the workplace with white supervisors or colleagues often described their experiences in ways that resembled "master and slave dynamics." They also tended to unnecessarily defer to white and *resentfully waited for white-others to give them opportunities*. This speaks to Wilson's (2009) theory that African Americans may paradoxically rely on the oppressor to undue oppression, which stems from a sense of helplessness that is deeply rooted in slavery.

Robinson (1995) and Young (2004) more positively conceptualized African Americans as facing their collective, grim reality and being adaptive enough to adopt a protective attitude that will help them survive mentally. Wilson (2009) and Parham et al. (1999) cautioned that *slave mentalities* may lead African-Americans to "resign" to what they perceive as the inevitability of their subservient position in white-dominated society, which can reinforce their traumatic helplessness. Similarly, Young (2004) studied African-American men who lived in inner city communities and found that they often felt trapped in overwhelming poverty and were powerless to change their lives. Similarly to Young (2004), Johnson (2002) noted that African-American men who are of lower socio-economic status often feel an inability to develop a positive view of their blackness, which Parham et al. (1999) noted to be *the key factor* in African American development and well-being.

Parham et al. (1999) noted that African Americans who experience traumatic helplessness are more likely to give up on becoming educated or successful in the workplace, which can help to liberate them from the traumatic effects of white racism. Parham et al. (1999) noted that, in this defeated state, African Americans may be more likely to behave in ways that are not true to their core, Afro-centric values. As an example, the authors describe African Americans who feel helpless as being more susceptible to criminal behavior and violating the Afro-centric principle: to attack another African American is to attack ones' self.

Alleyne (2004a) and Alleyne (2004b) noted that, for African-Americans, victim mentalities are a symptom of *internalized oppression*. Parham et al. (1999) elaborated that African Americans who have internalized white racism are predisposed to acting the oppression out in ways that increase rates of the social problems that are epidemics in the most notorious inner city African American communities. Like chronic physical abuse, internalized oppression correlates with health problems, domestic violence, depression, and PTSD (Lieberman et al., 2008; Briere et al., 2006; Gump, 2010; Walker, 2004; Alleyne, 2004a; Alleyne, 2004b; Robinson, 1995; Lum, 2003; Waites, 2004; Wilson, 2009). I have now demonstrated that interpersonal traumas increase risk for PTSD, and that white racism can be internalized and acted out in ways that are consistent with PTSD. This supported the theory that white racism meets criteria for a trauma for African Americans.

The difference in the black psychological discipline (as compared to the more mainstream trauma theories) is that the symptoms are considered symptoms of *systemic rather than psychic deficiency*. Whereas the trauma theories conceptualize interpersonal trauma as occurring in a more immediate environment (i.e. parent-child or intimate-partner relationships), the Afro-centric theories broaden the environment to include larger systemic forces like racism and poverty. I will now present Kozol's (2005) research on inner city African American public schools, which will be shown to illustrate this theory of larger systemic deficiency in lower income, urban African American communities.

Kozol (2005) found that the majority of public schools in lower-income, urban African American communities were woefully understaffed, poorly designed, and underfunded. These schools also operated on policies which were known by larger educational bureaucracies to be ineffective. For example, the author reported that African American children are known to learn more kinetically than traditionally, meaning that they benefit tremendously from opportunities to engage in creative expression, motion, and *doing*. Kozol (2005) emphasized that the arts, music, and other expressive arts classes stimulate areas of the brain that are vital to children's academic success. Kozol's (2005) points about African-American children's learning styles aligns with the Afro-centric values described by Parham et al. (1999).

Kozol (2005) noted that, despite the importance of these "electives"/expressive arts classes, when budget cuts became necessary at the schools under study, the arts classes were usually the first to go. They tended to be replaced by standardized testing and more rigorous disciplinary procedures on the grounds that these new policies were cost-effective. However, these policies tended not to exist in more affluent, predominantly white schools that were better funded and knowledgeable that such policies are not effective.

Kozol (2005) concluded that such disparaging realities naturally lead African-American public school students to feel alienated from the educational process. He elaborated that, contrary to popular stereotypes, a majority of them want to succeed and are encouraged to succeed by a majority of their parents. Similarly to Kozol's (2005) findings, Young (2001) qualitatively studied African-American men from inner city communities and found that (also contrary to popular stereotypes) most of them were goal-oriented, perceptive, and thoughtful; which is why they were also aware enough of white-dominated societies' barriers to their success to feel discouraged or saddened. The sum total of which supports the theory of systemic deficiency in African American communities, which is consistent with the theory that white racism is a traumatic threat that can be internalized and acted out in ways that parallel posttraumatic symptomology.

Discussion Question: *Re-consider the case of Joey that was presented in the previous chapter. Given what you have read about African Americans' history of oppression and research reports of how it manifests, how might Joey's presentation in therapy might have been influenced by historical and cultural factors?*

____

____

____

____

____

____

____

Now that I have discussed how (lower-income, urban) African-Americans may be affected by white racism, I will present a black psychological theory or how they can heal from its traumatic effects. Parham et al. (1999) stated that, in order for African Americans to heal, they need to stop blaming the system in ways that are not productive, hating whiteness, and waiting for white society to concede opportunities such as through more liberal social policy. The authors conceptualized these mentalities as recreating victimhood.

Parham et al. (1999) elaborated that, in order for African Americans to recover from their historically traumatic wounds, they need to develop a sense of security and positivity about their blackness. The authors defined positive ethnic identity for African Americans as a mature sense of comfort with one's own blackness and a critical consciousness of oppression. This involves a non-reactionary awareness of white racism and an ability to reflect on it and use the Afro-centric values and practices to repel its negative effects.

Discussion Question: *In your clinical work with African American clients, how might you help them develop what has been cited as a necessary critical race-consciousness? How might a white therapists' whiteness be both helpful AND/OR harmful in this respect?*

____

____

____

____

____

____

____

The difference between critical consciousness and the hyper sensitivity discussed previously is that, when African-Americans are critically conscious of their oppression, they feel internally secure about their blackness though without the reactionary vigilance to potentially racist threats. Parham et al.'s (1999) points about how African Americans can heal from their historically traumatic wounds by developing a more emotional sense of security and mental perspective parallels the emotional and mental goals of trauma treatment.

Gaylord-Harden et al. (2006) found that African American youth who had positive senses of ethnic identity experienced fewer symptoms of anxiety and depression than white youth, even though the African American youth under study endured more stressful life events. In that sense, positive ethnic identity may protect African Americans from some of the harmful effects of social inequalities.

The Black Psychological theory of African American racial identity development is rooted in *Nigresence theory* (Parham et al., 1999; Robinson, 1995). This theory operates from the premise that African Americans initially try to ingratiate themselves with the larger white-dominated society. At some point, they are confronted with the harsh reality that they will never be truly accepted and treated as equals by the racist mainstream. This realization initially feels shocking, and leads African Americans to become vehemently anti-white and sensationally pro-black. This sensationalism may be expressed through wearing distinctively African clothes, being very outspoken about racial issues, and more overtly and dramatically expressing pro-blackness. Despite the sensationalism, in this middle stage of identity development, African American are relatively insecure about their blackness (Parham et al., 1999). In the final, most mature stage of identity development, African Americans are more stable, secure, and modestly positive about their blackness; neither sensationalist nor ashamed, which parallels the trauma theory of constructing a new and more integrated narrative. Johnson (2002) validated Nigresence theory through *qualitative research*, which Jones (1982b) noted to be the preferred methodology for capturing the subtleties of African Americans' experiences.

In Haley's (1964) biography of Malcolm X, Malcolm is described as having gone through a process of ethnic identity development that coincides with the stages of Nigresence theory. In early adulthood, Malcolm X tended to "conk" his hair and otherwise behave in ways that suggested that he was trying to assimilate with white society. He eventually ended up in prison where he was mentored by an African American Muslim. Through this Muslim's guidance, Malcolm learned more about the historical plight of his people and came to realize that he, like other African Americans, would never be accepted and treated as equals by the racist majority. At this point, Malcolm became a more revolutionary spiritual mentor who spoke out publicly against white domination and encouraged African Americans to defend themselves against police brutality and other traumatic threats "by any means necessary." This is of course *the part* of Malcolm's story that tends to be the most sensationalized.

Haley (1964) transcribed that Malcolm X promoted violence and a more revolutionary spirit soon after being released from prison, which is consistent with my experiences with men who have recently been incarcerated for significant periods of time. Haley (1964) elaborated that, after Malcolm was back in the community for long enough to adjust prosocially, he was much calmer, less vehemently revolutionary, and was more interested in understanding the true, peaceful meaning of the Muslim faith. This interest inspired him to take the Muslim pilgrimage to Mecca where he was shocked to meet white-skinned Muslims who treated black-skinned Muslims as *social equals*. In America at that time in history, African Americans were winning various *political equalities*, though mainstream society remained largely reluctant to grant African Americans *social equality*. This latter sense of equality would have included equal access to education, employment, and housing. In the Middle East, Malcolm lived amongst white-skinned Muslims who regularly invited black-skinned Muslims to their homes, to eat with them, live amongst them, and communicate on more than superficial levels. In a micro-filmed lecture, Sue (2000) stated that such expressions of social equality are what will ultimately weaken the force of racism in contemporary society.

According to Haley (1964), after Malcolm returned to America from Mecca, he remained strongly pro-black and wary of white people becoming actively involved in his movement. Malcolm's concern was that white people would naturally take over the pro-black movement, which African Americans would naturally allow. Malcolm's concern is legitimized through research in support of the theory of internalized oppression. Nevertheless, when Malcolm returned from Mecca, he no longer advocated for African Americans to engage in violence, expressed remorse for his more reactionary refusal to work cooperatively with whiteswho were sensitive to his cause, and advocated for African Americans in a more mature, cooperative, and systemic way that is consistent with the contemporary community organizing strategies that are recommended by Waites (2004).

Doing Therapy with African American Clients

Thus far, I have presented a general theory of trauma and a black psychological theory of African American development as rooted in trauma. I will now talk more about how these historically-rooted traumas may manifest in barriers to therapeutic engagement when African Americans are paired with white therapists. I will then present therapy cases of African Americans which will illustrate some of these challenges and how these challenges can be worked through by orienting treatment to African Americans historically rooted survival strategies.

Parham et al. (1999) cautioned that African Americans are not a monolithic people and therefore cannot be treated clinically as if they are all the same. The authors also encouraged white therapists to more deeply consider pattern cross-cultural dynamics and orient treatment to align with afro-centric values. I take this point a step further in linking it to trauma theory, which provides a stronger base of evidence for the formulations of my cases. This is particularly important because one of the primary critiques of black psychology is that it has not been empirically supported by research.

This is important because African Americans (and lower income, urban African Americans in particular) are a historically underserved and highly at-risk population. In my experience, white therapists are far more readily available than African American therapists. Furthermore, Parham et al. (1999) cautioned that not all African American therapists are able to work constructively with African American clients because African American therapists may have their own unresolved issues with blackness. Thus, in order for African American clients to be more fully served, specific cross-cultural competencies for white therapists need to be developed; which will be the focus of the rest of this paper.

Reese (1998), Waites (2004), and Lum (2003) noted that African Americans' are often reluctant to engage in therapy. The authors explained that this relates to historically-rooted beliefs that one should solve one's own problems or at least solve them within one's own family and community. Lum (2003) and Parham et al. (1999) noted that African Americans seek professional help only when all other options have been exhausted and their presenting problems are sufficiently overwhelming. Adkins (2010) noted that African Americans often view the seeking of therapy as evidence of personal weakness and hurt pride. Lieberman et al. (2008) noted that, when African Americans do present for therapy, they often experience therapeutic engagement techniques as trickery.

Parham et al. (1999) noted that African Americans' barriers to therapeutic engagement are even more formidable when they are paired with white therapists. Lum (2003) noted this to be particularly true for lower income, urban African Americans. Jones' (1982) found that there is no significant difference in therapeutic outcome for African Americans who are paired with African American therapists *or* white therapists. Nevertheless, African American clients overwhelmingly prefer to work with African American therapists and up to 50% of them who are paired with a white therapist drop out after one session, usually because they don't feel understood and connected with (Parham et al., 1999; Duncan et al., 2007; African American Therapists, 2008).[1] It *may* be that just being in closer emotional proximity to whiteness triggers African-Americans' historically traumatic wounds, which activates the self-protective/survival strategies which may protect them in harsh surrounding environments *and* inhibit therapeutic engagement.

In my experience, it has been helpful to non-defensively acknowledge (to myself and in clinical supervision) that a majority of my lower income, urban African American clients do not engage with me as my white clients. When I sense the presence of barriers to therapeutic engagement in my work with African Americans, I often feel irritated. Through clinical supervision, I have unearthed that this dynamic brings up hard feelings about my not having being very accepted in my early life described in the beginning of this chapter.

[1] Africanamericantherapists.com is a professional list serve that is made up of clinicians who are committed to increasing the effectiveness of professional helping efforts with African American clients. This source regularly publishes scholarly material online, including the statistics noted in-text.

Discussion Question: *Describe a case where you had a strong emotional reaction to a client from a different racial or cultural background than you. Might there be any broader cross-cultural implications of what was happening? If so, please describe.*

____

____

____

____

____

____

____

I have sometimes been able to work through the irritation I described by considering that my lower income, urban African American client's reluctance to engage with me (and my irritable response) is potentially reminiscent of a historically traumatic dynamic. I have also found it helpful to reflect on my personal experiences of growing up in a lower income, urban African American community and remember that it was common knowledge that keeping one's mouth closed to authorities (including counselor types) was known to be necessary to prevent police or social service investigations, which usually lead to families being separated and men being incarcerated.

This reflection has sometimes lead me to re-frame what I instinctively considered to be my lower income, urban African American client's "resistance" to engaging with me as their best efforts to *resist oppression*. Robinson (1995) and (Benard (2004) described resistance as African Americans' core survival strategy throughout history and emphasized that it has been particularly necessary in lower income, urban African American communities where traumatic threats (such as police brutality) are more severe. Thus, because the threats are more severe, a predisposition to resist potentially oppressive forces is particularly necessary. The predisposition to resist could therefore be conceptualized as a symptom of trauma.

In session, I have found it helpful to think about my lower-income, urban African American client's resistance as expressions of *resilience*. Benard (2004) described resilience as a developmental capacity to adapt and survive through harsh surrounding circumstances by *resisting* threats to homeostasis. The author elaborates that clients of color demonstrate resilience when they resist potentially oppressive threats. I have found that a resilience-oriented therapeutic approach has helped to turn my irritation (about engagement barriers) into empathy, which of course helps to build relationships. This discussion supports Jones' (1982b) conclusion that empathy and counter transference are the two key factors in the psychotherapeutic experiences of African Americans who are paired with white therapists.

It is also important to note that the theory of resilience has been tested and validated in relevant research studies. Markstrom et al. (1997) found that there was a correlation between resilience and *ego strength*, which was noted by Markstrom and Kalmanir (2001) to have a relationship with *positive ethnic identity for African-Americans,* which was described in the previous section as a strong correlate of African American wellness. The relationship between resilience and positive ethnic identity for African Americans may suggest that a resilience-oriented therapeutic approach can help African Americans develop more positive ethnic identities. This is doubly important because it provides white therapists with a less presumptuous way to orient therapy to afro-centric values.

In addition to their core strength of resisting oppression, African Americans have other historically-rooted strengths and survival strategies which I have sometimes acknowledged directly and intuitively made use of in extended family (Waites, 2004; Lum, 2003; Logan, 2001). Lum (2003) described these strengths as rooted in the African tradition of clanship. The author elaborated that these strengths helped African Americans survive through slavery and remain primary coping strategies in present-day, African American communities. These strengths have been noted by many authors to insulate African Americans from the harmful effects of stress, poverty, depression, and traumatic oppression (Gaylord-Harden et al., 2006; Alleyne, 2004a; Alleyne, 2004b; Waites, 2004; Parham et al., 1999; Sharpe, 2010; Michalopoulus et al., 2009; Grant, 2010; Lum, 2003; Robinson, 1995; Stewert et al., 2006). This discussion of how African-Americans' may use group-oriented and community-oriented survival strategies to protect themselves from traumatic threats parallels my previous discussion about how social support can help chronic trauma survivors stabilize and recover from their traumas. This parallel is important because it shows that the linkage between African American's common plight and the core principles of trauma theory extends into their recovery process.

I will now present brief case vignettes which demonstrate what this has sometimes looked like in practice. The first case I will talk about is my ongoing individual work with a 25 year old African-American male who has lived in an impoverished inner city community throughout his whole life. He has been in therapy with me for two years. He has been a gang member since he was 15, was raised by an alcoholic mother, never knew his father, and suffers from a severe psychotic disorder.

Discussion Question: *What might you be feeling if you were beginning to work with this client and how might your reactions be harmful* <u>*and/or*</u> *informative to the therapy?*

____

____

____

____

____

He presents as very intelligent, but with a strong tendency to intellectualize his feelings and speak at length about his psychosis-laden philosophies about life. This usually annoys me. When he is in a therapy group that I facilitate, I have noticed that other clients in the group seem to feel annoyed for similar reasons when he speaks in this manner.

I have sometimes calmed my annoyance by thinking about how, at a very unconscious level, he may be trying to push people away for fear they might hurt or abandon him. This coincides with my previous discussion about how trauma may shatter the survivor's basic sense of trust and how African Americans' may instinctively resist oppressive threats.

While thinking about this client in this more empathic way, I have sometimes interrupted his lengthy disclosures to ask him if he is feeling somehow unsafe or threatened and is therefore speaking in broader, more general terms in order to protect himself. Usually, he readily agrees, calms down, and goes emotionally deeper into what he is afraid of. This is an example of how to reframe resistance in a way that meets a trauma-survivor's needs for trust and safety.

The second case I will discuss is my therapeutic work with an African-American man who I worked with a few years ago when I was a counselor in a residential treatment center for men who had recently been released from prison. This client was in his 40's and had been incarcerated for the last 30 years of his life. He told me he was most recently in prison for kidnapping, though he did not volunteer details of what happened. I decided not to ask for details because I was concerned that doing so might increase his resistance.

Discussion Question: *What reactions might you be having to this client if you were beginning to work with him? Might your reactions potentially have any broader cultural-historical implications? If so, please discuss.*

Early in our therapeutic work, I told him that I had never been to prison and asked him what it was like, though disclaimers that I would understand if he didn't want to talk about it. Over the next two months of our work together, he told me about how the guards used to strip him naked and lock him in solitary confinement for days at a time without food. Somehow, I knew the guards were white.

When this man would tell me about his oppressive experiences in prison, he would often watch me closely as if monitoring my reactions. I remember feeling shocked and horrified by what he had to go through and wondered if my feelings were a microcosm of what he felt. I also felt a strong urge to somehow take care of him. Somehow, I think he knew that I understood as much as I possibly could. Meanwhile, he was doing well in treatment. He did not have any significant conflicts with other clients, passed several random drug tests, and regularly attended therapy groups and other treatment functions.

Then, almost suddenly, other clients started to get angry with him for stealing and he failed a drug test. I responded to his misbehaviors by scolding him sternly. This approach was encouraged by my treatment center. Additionally, I have found that I have sometimes needed to have a harder, clinical edge in order to be taken seriously by a hardened, criminal justice-referred population of color; particularly as a younger, white male clinician. I also remember reacting to my client of frustration, which led him to avoid contact with me. Two weeks later, he was back in prison.

My client's behavior in treatment suggested that he was profoundly affected by long term institutionalization. It would be unrealistic to think that I could treat 20 years of such conditioning in just three months. Nevertheless, I can't help but to think that, in the beginning of our work, maybe he was testing me by telling me about how hard his life had been. I might have passed this first test, which might be why our relationship began to develop. Then, at a very unconscious level, he may have acted out more severely and succeeded in recreating traumatic dynamics in our relationship.

Discussion: *Describe a time when your emotional reactions to an oppressed client either damaged your developing therapeutic relationship, or at least could have damaged it.*

____

____

____

____

____

____

____

LIMITATIONS

The primary limitation of this chapter is that *a white male* is writing about African Americans. Though I have personal experience in a lower-income, urban African American community, my not being African American makes it inherently problematic for me to write about African Americans. Furthermore, my home community is not necessarily representative of all other African American communities. Therefore, although my personal experiences are relevant to the topic, they may not be entirely generalizeable.

It is also important to note that this chapter leans in the direction of universalizing African Americans' experiences. Thus, the paper risks Parham et al.'s (1999) noted *ghetto-ization* of African American culture. Jones (1982b, 1984) expressed a similar concern about how universalizing the experiences of African Americans' deprives them of their individuality, which re-creates the oppression that is at the core of their traumatic suffering. Contrastingly, Parham et al. (1999)

Jones (1982b; 1984) agrees with Parham et al. (1999) on the point that white therapists need to address their personal issues with blackness and be open to *African Americans' uniquely African American experiences*. However, the latter authors' seemed dubious about the possibility that white therapists could learn about the afro-centric values and apply them to clinical practice without reinforcing racist stereotypes. It is important to note that Jones' (1982b) conclusions were based on the results of massive qualitative study of African American's experiences in psychotherapy and how those experiences were affected by therapeutic matching. Thus, the authors' conclusions were strongly supported by research.

Though I believe that I have piloted a culturally sensitive and informative theory, further study is needed in order to establish validity and reliability.

CONCLUSION

In summary, I first presented a more general theory of trauma and posttraumatic symptom development. I then showed that white racism may act as a trauma trigger for African Americans and may affect African-Americans in ways that parallel the effects of chronic interpersonal trauma. I proceeded to show how white racism may influence African American's development and psychotherapeutic experiences with white American therapists in ways that coincide with the core principles of trauma theory. It is also important to mention that the same core survival strategies that have helped African Americans survive throughout their history of traumatic oppression continue to help them survive in harsh surrounding environments *and/or increase rates of social problems in their communities*, and can also inhibit therapeutic engagement *and/or be called upon to work through historically-rooted engagement barriers*.

Writing this chapter involved as introspection about my own experiences as intellectually-natured research. In my experience, this deeper self-examination has been absolutely vital to working as competently and sensitively with African American clients as possible, as a white therapist. I would expect this kind of introspection to be necessary for other white therapists to work competently with African Americans, which is consistent with the recommendations of Sue and Sue (2008). My experience has also been that white therapists tend to be uncomfortable with such deeper, cross-culturally focused exploration, which is typically expressed through denial, liberalization, or intellectualization. Parham et al. (1999) noted that deeper, fearless exploration is an absolutely necessary step in the direction of competently serving African American clients; the absence of which contributes to their ongoing suffering.

Chapter 4

DILEMMAS IN THE TREATMENT OF BORDERLINE PERSONALITY DISORDER

Graham Danzer and Simon Ferber

INTRODUCTION

I have noticed an ongoing debate in clinical circles about whether clients who present for psychotherapy should be diagnosed and then treated clinically based on what tends to work for similarly diagnosed clients or if clients should be treated clinically based on the therapist's assessment of their emotional needs as individuals. Though these two ways of working clinically are not necessarily mutually exclusive, a majority of therapists that I have interacted with tend to be more strongly oriented towards the more diagnostic therapeutic approach *or* the emotionally nearer, client-centered approach.

I will explore this dilemma of approaches by presenting the dialectical behavior therapeutic approach to treating borderlines; which emphasizes both a skills-focused approach to treating symptoms *and* the emotionally nearer therapeutic principle of validation. Then, I will present the case of *Teresa* (who meets criteria for borderline personality disorder) and discuss how she responded when I intuitively validated her emotional experiences and how she responded when I intuitively tried to help her develop skills and apply those skills to her various challenges. Thus, the two core operating principles of DBT will be shown to be a microcosm of my aforementioned dilemma of approaches; both in theory and in practice. My hope is that this paper will raise awareness of the importance of my core subject matter, which I am seeing as critically relevant to clinical practice and yet rarely researched.

BORDERLINE PERSONALITY DISORDER

It is important to first define a personality disorder, which I will do by presenting Sperry's (1995) theory of personality disorders and how *personality disorders* differ from more functional *personalities*. Then, I will present Sperry's more diagnostic conceptualization of borderline personality disorder *and* an attachment theory of borderline personality disorder.

These two frameworks will provide an illustration of each side of my aforementioned dilemma of therapeutic approaches.

Sperry (1995) defines the human personality as a cluster of various *personality characteristics* which give people their senses of individuality. These characteristics include sense of humor, primary defensive strategies, degree of assertiveness, temperament, and degree of autonomy versus dependence.

Sperry (1995) theorizes that the cluster of most people's personality characteristics tend to fit into various *personality styles.* So long as the personality characteristics (of the personality style) are used flexibly, with discretion, and in relative moderation, they are positive attributes which will help people achieve success in otherwise challenging areas of life.

Sperry (1995) explains that these personality characteristics become symptoms of a personality disorder when they take more extreme forms, or are used rigidly and without discretion. The author elaborates that this sense of extremity and rigidity makes it difficult for personality disordered individuals to negotiate relationships with a majority of others (who will usually have more flexible and moderate personalities). This discrepancy usually leads to considerable problems in personality disordered individuals' relationships, which is one of the primary reasons why many personality disordered individuals are more socially isolated than they really want to be (Sperry, 1995). In follow up research, Sperry (2003) maintains his conceptualization of personality as operating on a spectrum that ranges from healthy to pathological. Where the individual lies on the personality spectrum depends on the relative degree of prominence and extremity of the personality characteristics noted in Sperry (1993).

Sperry (1995) describes one with the borderline *personality style* as being dynamic, flexible, creative, and charming; which often leads to emotionally deep relationships. The borderline *personality disorder* is evidenced by a more profoundly unstable and fragmented self-image which is expressed emotionally through chronic feelings of emptiness and deep-seated fears of abandonment. Whereas an individual with the borderline personality style can flexibly adjust in interpersonal exchanges in order to support and maintain relationships, individuals with borderline personality disorder will often behave seductively, self-mutilate, and shift rapidly from idealizing others to devaluing them in effort to achieve complete enmeshment.

Such chaotic behavior will often repel borderline personality disorder individuals caring others, which may trigger their fears of abandonment and lead them to respond ragefully, with affective instability, or to decompensate emotionally. Sperry (1995) noted that borderlines typically try to regulate this intense emotionality through suicidal or para-suicidal behavior, drug and alcohol abuse, and high-risk sexual behavior. Such high risk behaviors often lead borderlines to cycle in and out of hospitals and treatment centers where they often pull (typically undertrained and poorly supervised) inpatient staff into highly complex and problematic transference and counter transference dyads; which often lead to overly behavioral, confrontational, and punitive treatments, which results in poor treatment outcomes and high rates of clinician burn-out (Eastwick et al., 2005; Livesley, 2005; Turbott, 2004).

Discussion Question: *Consider your therapeutic work with clients from disenfranchised backgrounds who may have met criteria for a personality disorder, or what it might be like to work therapeutically with a client-of-color who met criteria for a personality disorder. How* *might thinking about the client as having a personality disorder been helpful to treatment* and/or *harmful to the therapeutic relationship?*

In the last few paragraphs, I presented a more medical modular/diagnostic conceptualization of borderline pathology. I will now present an attachment theory of this disorder, which I have found to be a more helpful to think about borderlines as I work with them clinically. I have found this way of thinking to be helpful to the therapeutic work because it helps me to have empathy for them, which aids in the development of a relationship. This is consistent with Sperry's (2003) theory of a better treatment prognosis (for personality disordered individuals in general and borderlines in particular) when there is less of an emphasis on temperament and biological factors, and more consideration of more relationally-oriented factors like trauma, early life attachment experiences, and adult attachment style.

Whereas Sperry's (1993) earlier conceptualization of borderlines was more pathologically oriented, Gregory (2004) describes borderlines as trying to soothe themselves or at least distract themselves from painful emotions by trying to become enmeshed with idealized mother figures. The author elaborates that borderlines do this because they typically come from families where only extremes brought about vitally necessary changes. Furthermore, their mothers typically did not provide them with the nurturing and mirroring which would have built a more secure attachment system, which would normally help more securely and flexibly charactered people manage their emotions (Diamond et al., 2003; Bateman et al., 2003). Similarly, Eastwick et al. (2005) noted that borderline pathology largely stems from negative childhood experiences, which damaged borderlines' abilities to process information and maintain healthier self-images, and perpetuates their maladaptive belief systems. Similarly to Eastwick et al. (2005), Linehan (1993a) noted that borderlines tend to have severe histories of trauma and maltreatment in early life *and* lack the cognitive abilities that would normally facilitate more secure and functional relational behavior. The research in this last paragraph is important because it shows that borderline pathology is ultimately related to *attachment* (Bateman et al., 2003; Diamond et al., 2003). The authors elaborate that a more empathic way to conceptualize borderlines' often chaotic relational behavior is to think about it as *disorganized attachment* behavior, which I will now illustrate through an attachment theory of borderlines' suicidal and para-suicidal behavior. This is important for my discussion because it is an example of how even the most severe symptomology can be conceptualized in a more relational way.

Linehan et al. (1991) describe borderlines as self-injuring or emotionally de-compensating in order to ask others for support. Linehan (1993a) emphasizes that self-injury is not a typical cry for help, but that it is a less adaptive coping skill that stems from weaker cognitive functioning and a weak social support system.

Borderlines' self-injurious behavior is often labeled as *manipulation*, though this label doesn't fit because the definition of manipulation is to shrewdly or artfully manage difficult situations (Linehan, 1993a). In contrast, borderlines tend to be much more forceful, direct, and unskillful in their demands of others. Furthermore, although their self-injurious and para-suicidal behavior often brings people into proximity, it is not suggestive of lying or manipulation. Rather, it is an expression of ambivalence about living and of deep-seated emptiness and emotional pain.

Linehan (1993a) also emphasizes that borderlines' more extreme relational behaviors are not indicative of their being *needy;* as is often assumed. Rather, borderlines have understandably strong emotional reactions to having the emotional support of potentially caring others rationed to them. For example, their contacts with clinicians tend to be fairly short. Additionally, my experience has been that borderlines' attachment figures tend to be able to only tolerate borderlines for so long before necessarily needing emotional and physical space from them.

Linehan (1993a) elaborates that this deprivation naturally leads borderlines to protest in ways that would be considered acceptable and understandable if it were a cancer patient being denied medical care. The author contends that the only real difference is that the source of borderlines' sickness is mental *rather than physical,* though their reaction to being emotionally deprived is normal and healthy because attachment is vitally necessary to physical survival (Bowlby 1960; 1963; 1969). As discussed previously, Bowlby found that infants that were sufficiently emotionally deprived did not survive regardless of having their basic physical needs met. Thus, borderlines' protesting what they experience as emotional deprivation is ultimately both an emotional *and* a physical survival strategy.

For example, my experience has been that, when borderlines threaten suicide or self-mutilate, clinicians and family members often engage in a flurry of problem solving-oriented activity and tend to remain mentally preoccupied with and in closer physical proximity to the borderline long after the borderlines' more immediate crises' have been resolved. In that sense, borderlines' (albeit highly disorganized) attachment behavior creates a significant degree of the emotional or physical proximity that they so deeply desire and is vital to all people's emotional survival (Beck et al., 2004).

The problem is that the attention that is generated by borderline pathology tends to be overwhelmingly negative. This is also true for borderlines experiences with their therapists; which makes the management of the therapist's counter transference a top priority (Linehan et al., 1991).

Therapeutic Strategy for Working with Borderlines

Now that I have presented both a more diagnostic and a more relational conceptualization of borderline pathology, I will talk more about treatment strategy. In this section, I will present the basic operating principles of the therapeutic relationship that make a more positive treatment prognosis possible for this population. Then, in my next section, I will move into the cognitive modular approaches to treating the pathology, including DBT, and talk more specifically about interventions. This particular order is important because, in my experience, a more client-centered, relationally-oriented way of thinking about and responding to borderlines makes the interventions more likely to be effective.

Borderlines' history of overwhelmingly poor treatment outcomes inspired Marsha Linehan (et al., 1991; 1993a; 1993b) to become particularly interested in treating them. Linehan (1993a) describes this professional interest as developing when she worked on a CBT-oriented treatment team that observed her and took notes on her clinical practice with borderlines. The primary purpose of this research was to identify and make note of helpful interventions. Though intending to practice CBT, Linehan found herself instinctively moving back and forth from a more gentle empathy to irreverent confrontation. Later, she envisioned this *dialectic* as occurring on a teeter-totter with the therapist on one side and the client on the other. On some level, each was trying to *meet in the middle so that neither fell off*. This was Linehan's conceptualization of what happened as the therapist and client negotiated the emotional core of the therapeutic relationship.

From her research, Linehan's (1993a; 1993b) concluded that the borderline's therapist needed to be able to set and maintain necessary therapeutic boundaries, but to also be flexible, nurturing, patient, non-personalizing, and able to operate with discretion (Krawitz and Watson, 2000). This would provide the borderline with the emotionally close relationship that he or she so desperately wanted, though in a way that reinforced that emotional closeness could occur *safely* (Bateman et al., 2003; Diamond et al., 2003). Gregory (2004) and Livesley (2005) researched borderlines' experiences in therapy and validated these theories that were originally advanced by Linehan (et al., 1991; 1993a; 1993b).

In order to facilitate this more secure, emotionally close relationship with borderlines, several authors recommend that therapists engage in professional risk taking such as professionally self-disclosing and paradoxical interventions (Hayes et al., 2004; Linehan et al., 2002; Krawitz et al., 2004). The authors elaborate that this can help borderlines see the personhood of their therapists, which will help them *differentiate* and *mentalize*. Bateman et al. (2003) and Diamond et al. (2003) elaborate that these are core relational capacities that borderlines typically lack (because they were emotionally deprived in early life) and need to build through a secure attachment-connection to the therapist. Gregory (2004) elaborates that, if the therapist can consistently and reliably operate as the borderlines' benevolent parental figure, the borderline will begin to develop properly, which means eventually switching from seeing the therapist as an idealized mother figure (who should be enmeshed with) to seeing the therapist as a strong parental figure. The author elaborates this will help borderlines internalize the positive attributes of their therapists, which will help them overcome their fears and strengthen their egos. Whereas borderlines were once historically lumped together as hopeless cases, more relationally-oriented approaches that considered attachment factors have led to far more positive treatment prognosis' (Linehan, 1993b; Sperry, 2003).

With these aforementioned relational principles in mind, Linehan (1993a; 1993b) sought to develop a therapeutic model that could help borderlines *manage themselves* in times of emotional crisis. She strongly believed that they need to be responsible for their own treatment and behavior outside of therapy.

This was important because, before Linehan, borderlines were often treated clinically based on analytic or behaviorally-oriented approaches, which Linehan conceptualized as putting the onus of the responsibility on the therapist to either resolve the client's inner conflict or re-structure the client's environment (Linehan et al., 1991; 1993a; 1993b).

Linehan's research reflects an appreciation of the behaviorist's fundamental goal for clients to learn more functional behaviors and an appreciation for the analytic goal for clients to work through painful emotions. Linehan's writings also more positively viewed borderlines as not necessarily needing the longer term, insight-oriented therapeutic work (that was recommended by the psychoanalysts) nor the excessively structured environment (that is often recommended by more behaviorally-focused clinicians) in order to increase functional behavior.

Linehan (1991; 1993a; 1993b) concurred with the analysts' position on borderlines needing significant therapeutic contact and emotional closeness in the therapeutic relationship. She also concurred with the behaviorists' position on borderlines needing a more positively stimulating and containing environment. She then hypothesized that these treatment goals could be addressed through a therapy that allowed for significant therapeutic contact that was gently and empathically oriented towards helping borderlines develop skills that could help them emotionally regulate and communicate effectively. Linehan (1993b) elaborated that, if borderlines were trained in therapy to use these skills outside of therapy, they would be better prepared to call upon those skills in times of distress in order to resolve (or at least modulate) internal-emotional or interpersonal conflicts. The end result would be that borderlines would be more mentally equipped to manage their emotions and resolve their interpersonal-environmental challenges rather than necessarily depending on a superior other to solve their problems for them.

THE DEVELOPMENT OF DIALECTICAL BEHAVIOR THERAPY

Linehan's therapeutic strategy for working with borderlines comes right out of Aaron Beck's *cognitive therapy*, which eventually influenced the development of *cognitive behavioral therapy,* which then influenced the development of Linehan's *dialectical behavior therapy*. I will now present what is essentially an evolution of these cognitively-oriented theories.

Beck (1973) developed his cognitive model after having grown sufficiently dissatisfied with the behaviorist and psychoanalytic approaches. Beck (1973) disagreed with the behaviorists' view that (positive or negative) stimulus in the environment mentally conditions people to the point that behavior is predictable. He also disagreed with the psycho-analysts' view of emotional discomfort as being so deeply rooted in earlier life conflicts. Beck's primary concern about each of the aforementioned theories was that they both conceptualized the inter-psychic roots of human suffering as deeply rooted in the unconscious.

He concurred with the psychoanalyst's position on patients being caught in dysfunctional inter-psychic patterns which increased their emotional suffering. He also agreed with the behaviorist's position on how these dysfunctional inter-psychic patterns were influenced by dysfunctional interchanges in their surrounding environments.

Beck (1973) added that patients tend to *think* about their inter-psychic and externally-oriented conflicts in ways that increase their suffering. Beck observed that patients tended to fall into distinct patterns of distorted thinking, including making erroneous assumptions and misinterpreting the meaning of significant life events. He observed that patients often take their distorted cognitions as facts, which increased emotional suffering, which fueled impulsive behavior, which lead to more problems, which then increased emotional suffering even more.

Unlike the psychoanalysts and behaviorists, Beck (1973) more positively conceptualized the mental contribution to human suffering and the key to correcting it as operating at a level that is much closer to consciousness. Beck (1973) believed that therapy could help patients become more aware of the patterns in their distorted thinking, and that this increase in self-awareness would help them catch their distorted thoughts *in the act* outside of therapy. He anticipated that this increase in mental awareness would inhibit the flow of negative emotions that would normally fuel impulsive behavior. Thus, Beck saw emotional suffering and dysfunctional behavior as *mentally correctable*. More recently, Beck et al. (2004) validated the efficacy of this cognitive theory through modern research methodologies.

I have often heard relational therapists critique cognitive therapies on the grounds that they underemphasize emotional and relational factors. However, Beck (1973) stresses that, in the beginning stages of therapy, the cognitive therapist should only seek to better understand and assess the patient's world view by asking questions about when various problems started, how the problems have developed, and how the patient feels about his or her problems. Beck (1973) strongly recommends that the therapist should not attempt to challenge the patient's faulty ways of thinking until the therapeutic relationship has developed to the point that the patient fully understands the good nature of the therapists' intentions. This shows that Beck (1973), the founder of the cognitive discipline, paid attention to emotional and relational factors.

In fact, integrating Beck's theory with the more traditionally analytic considerations of how earlier life conflicts influence the development of personality and influence what is happening in the therapeutic relationship forms the theoretical basis of *cognitive behavioral therapy* (Dobson, 2001). This approach builds on Albert Ellis' *rational-emotive behavior therapy (REBT)* and takes the traditionally analytic theory of defenses a step further in a more behaviorally-focused direction. Whereas analysts essentially conceptualize people as avoiding emotionally painful stimulus through *defensive mental processes*, the cognitive-behaviorists add that people may *physically* avoid emotionally painful stimulus through what is essentially *defensive behavior* (Dobson, 2001; Linehan, 1993a). The cognitive-behaviorists also integrated the behaviorists' emphasis on environmental conditioning by introducing positive rewards as strategies for increasing client's functional behavior (Dobson, 2001; Linehan, 1993a).

Thus, the cognitive-behavioral approach integrates what are traditionally analytic, behavioral, and cognitive therapeutic principles. *CBT* conceptualizes thoughts, feelings, and behavior as points on a triangle and gives credence to each model by emphasizing that intervention at any one of the three points on the triangle has the potential to positively affect the human processes on the other two points (Dobson, 2001).

Discussion Question: *Consider your own therapeutic work with clients-of-color. What are some of the cognitively-focused interventions that you have tried more than once (e.g. clarifying choices, encouraging alternate points of view, giving homework assignments, helping clients problem solve) ?Which cognitive interventions that you have repeatedly used seemed the most and least helpful to your clients, and why?*

Linehan integrated some of these core principles of CBT with eastern philosophical teachings to form *Dialectical Behavior Therapy* (Hayes et al., 2004). Linehan (1993a) defines DBT as an application of a broad array of cognitive and behavioral techniques; including assessment, collecting data on behavior, developing a collaborative working relationship, problem solving, exposure techniques, skills training, contingency management, and cognitive modification.

Linehan (1993a) defines the primary "dialectic" as: "the reconciliation of opposites in a continual process of synthesis" (p.19), which means accepting patients as they are, though also trying to help them change through both supportive and confrontative strategies. She particularly appreciated eastern teachings on *mindfulness*, which emphasize noticing one's emotions and witnessing what is happening inside of one's self without trying to change it. The author hypothesized that mindfulness training can help clients accept even their uncomfortable feelings as part of their humaneness, which would put those painful feelings in Beck's (1973) noted competent and realistic perspective, which would allow the feelings to pass rather than fueling impulsive behavior (Hayes et al., 2004). Thus, whereas Beck (1973) viewed emotional suffering and impulsive behavior as mentally *correctable,* Linehan viewed emotional suffering and impulsive behavior as mentally *manageable*. This last point speaks to the DBT principle of *distress tolerance,* which Linehan (1993a) defines as learning to bear pain skillfully.

Linehan's (1993a; 1993b) primary departure from Beck (1973) was that she recommended that therapy help client's learn acceptance of themselves rather than correcting their distorted thoughts and therefore necessarily *judging* them as bad. Hayes et al. (2004) emphasize that judgment of painful emotions heightens emotional suffering, which may fuel impulsive behavior. Linehan (1993a; 1993b) viewed that the therapist's primary strategy for helping clients learn acceptance is for the therapist to radically accept and *validate* all parts of the client's personhood, which would help clients feel better and therefore be more capable of making good decisions about how to respond appropriately to their emotional distress. The author defines validation as finding the wisdom in the client's statements and communicating understanding of that wisdom back to the client. Thus, Linehan (1993a; 1993b) recommended a more validating, less systematic approach to cognitive modification than what is typical in cognitive-behavioral therapeutic treatment.

Linehan (1993a) emphasizes that validation, acceptance, and attentiveness to therapy-interfering behaviors (which parallels transference and counter transference) are DBT-oriented *strategies for building a therapeutic relationship*. She elaborates that this marks an important progression from the earlier cognitive theories, which paid attention to relational factors, though said very little about *how to build a relationship.*

Linehan's (1993b) dialectical behavior therapeutic approach involves four distinct skills-focused modules, which include training on mindfulness, distress tolerance, emotional regulation, and *interpersonal effectiveness*; which would be particularly helpful for borderlines. The author more positively conceptualizes borderlines as already having the interpersonal skills that could help them necessarily: make requests of others, say no, advocate for themselves with others in ways that maintain self-esteem, avoid conflicts, and communicate their needs. She elaborated that the problem for borderlines is that their responses are most often guided by their fears, anxieties, and judgments, which interfere with their abilities to turn potentially confrontative interchanges in relationships into positive interchanges. Thus, the mindfulness and distress tolerance modules necessarily precede the interpersonal skills training because these first modules allow for the emotional grounding and regulation that make more effective communication possible.

Research on DBT supports that it is an effective treatment for reducing borderlines' self-injurious behavior and reducing the frequency and duration of their inpatient psychiatric hospital visits (Linehan, 1993a; 1993b). Neacsiu et al. (2010) found that DBT skills training increased borderlines' use of DBT skills, and that increased usage of DBT skills decreased depressive symptoms and suicidal gestures, and helped borderlines manage their anger.

Beck et al. (2004) expressed concern about how, although borderlines' caring others often report that DBT seems to help them *behave* better, borderlines themselves often report that the treatment doesn't help them *feel* better. Sperry (1995) cautions that borderlines may self-report feeling worse when they are behaving better because they fear that, if they get better, their therapists will abandon them. My experience has been that such insecurities (which are often labeled as manipulation) tend to evoke strong counter transference reactions in their therapists, which can make it difficult for therapists to provide borderlines with the warmth and radical acceptance that is noted by Linehan (1993a; 1993b) to be essential for their treatment.

My experience with borderlines has been that, regardless of their tendencies to be poor historians, *they need to be believed anyway* in order for their treatment to have the greatest healing potential. Livesley (2005) emphasizes that, if the therapist is consistently doubtful or suspicious, the therapy has the potential to recreate the same invalidating environment that the borderline typically comes from and is likely to lead to a poor therapeutic outcome. Linehan (1993b) similarly contends that borderlines tend to function well in positive and supportive relationships and to struggle in relationships that are invalidating; *including in therapy.* Sperry's (2003) more recent research similarly notes a more positive treatment prognosis for borderlines when the treatment is more holistic, relational, and considerate of attachment factors.

Discussion Question: *Think back to the case of the formerly incarcerated African-American man who was discussed in the last chapter. From a DBT perspective, what was the necessary therapeutic response to his various problematic behaviors? Would this approach be easy or difficult for you to implement in those circumstances, and why?*

These last paragraphs demonstrate that it is not only difficult to clinically treat borderlines, but that it is also difficult to evaluate the results of the treatment and even decide on criteria for evaluating the results. I will now present Teresa's case as an illustration of these challenges and how I have intuitively tried to work through them in ways that coincide with some of the aforementioned therapeutic principles. I will include some of my reflections that came up as I was working with her and then theorize about what was happening in our work in more depth in my discussion section.

TERESA

When I first met Teresa, I noticed that she was very beautiful, though also very sad. She was a darker skinned Latina in her early 20's, with freckles, long, curly brown hair, and deeply set eyes. She also stared down through the floor as if she felt completely hopeless.

Her sadness was so profound that it overwhelmed me. I was immediately wishing that I could help her, though I doubted I could, which lead me to feel even more anxious. Outside of my clinical work, I tend to be uncomfortable with sadness and powerlessness, which may be why I felt anxious when Teresa was so sad and powerless. This was what it was like during the first 15 minutes of our first session.

Then, I was almost relieved to remember that I had to ask her a series of intake questions. In my personal life, *doing things* often helps me focus my anxiety in productive ways. Though I didn't notice it at the time, I remember fairly rushing through the intake questions as if I was trying to get the whole thing over with as quickly and as painlessly as possible.

In answer to my questions, Teresa informed me that she had been mandatorily referred to my county mental health clinic by her county welfare worker. She said that she was referred after she repeatedly showed up late or did not show up at all to the welfare-to-work training program that she was required to attend in order to receive general assistance benefits. She added that, when she did show up to the training program, she was unable to concentrate and would suddenly start crying uncontrollably without knowing why. Several months of this led Teresa's welfare worker to insist that she come to my clinic for a mental health assessment.

Teresa told me about these experiences in a kind of frantic and pressured way. To me, it felt like she was almost demanding to know what was wrong with her. She expressed this desire to know by repeatedly asking, "why does this keep happening?!?! " By "this," she was referring to her various internal-emotional crises'.

In the moment, I took her questions literally. Over the next half an hour, I joined her in exploring possible causes of her problems and possible solutions to them. I asked a lot of assessment-style questions, such as when her problems started, when they tended to increase in severity, and what helped her manage herself in times of emotional crisis. Each question that I asked Teresa seemed to lead her to more frantically search for answers to what was troubling her. We also discussed her unsuccessful efforts to: get stable on psychiatric medications, engage in alternative therapies, and to work through painful emotions by utilizing self-care practices such as meditation and progressive relaxation.

During this discussion, Teresa informed me that she had been hospitalized for psychiatric reasons at least 10 times, though she changed the subject when I asked her about why she was hospitalized. I sensed that it would be better for the development of our relationship to assume that she might tell me the details of her hospitalizations at some point in the future if I really needed to know them.

Meanwhile, we were about a half an hour into our first session and none of our various problem solving efforts seemed to be helping Teresa find the sense of resolution she seemed to be looking for. In fact, Teresa always seemed to have two objections to every possible solution to her various life-problems that came up in-session. For example, when discussing her strained relationships with her family members, she began to consider different ways that she could speak up to them about her concerns. Then, she would immediately dismiss her efforts as pointless because her family members would not listen to her.

Discussion Question: *If you were Teresa's therapist, at this point in the therapy, what emotional reactions might you be having to Teresa and why? How might your reactions be helpful* <u>*and/or*</u> *harmful to your therapeutic work with her?*

____

____

____

The hopelessness of it all seemed to make Teresa feel even more anxious, which lead me to feel more anxious as well. It was as if the harder we tried to assess and solve her problems, the further away we got from any real sense of resolution, which demanded that we try harder to come up with solutions, which only drove us even further away.

By the end of the session, I felt pulled apart. For a brief moment, I reflected on some of the things Teresa had told me in the midst of her anxious flurries and my efforts to help her problem solve. She told me that she had been molested by a neighbor when she was six, had been in a physically abusive relationship in her teenage years, and had a mentally ill mother who refused psychiatric care and tended to be in and out of her life.

I felt a compelling need to take emotional care of Teresa, but the doubt that I could help her spoke louder. I let her know that weekly individual therapy might be helpful to her and inquired about whether she might be interested in meeting with a female therapist. I suggested that another woman might be better able to help her explore her various traumas, which might help her heal (from the traumas) and move on with her life.

Teresa vehemently opposed my suggestion on the basis that all women were back stabbing, gossiping, and otherwise untrustworthy. Looking back on it, this harsh view of women may have stemmed from her negative experiences with her mother.

Nevertheless, I could sense that Teresa wanted to come back to meet with me, which I found encouraging. I liked her and felt strongly sorrowful that she had such a hard life. The overwhelm that remained in the therapeutic room was immense, but I resolved myself to do what was in my power to help Teresa find the solutions to her problems that she seemed to be seeking. She agreed to come back to see me next week.

When she arrived at my office for our next session, I was quite surprised and uncomfortable to see that she was more ornately attired and barely contained in a very small blouse. I made a considerable effort to look away, though I tried not to look like I was looking away. I was concerned about reinforcing a sexualized dynamic that Teresa seemed to be pulling for, which might be detrimental to her self-esteem. I was also concerned that responding to her in an overly uncomfortable, excessively boundaried kind of way might make her feel ashamed. I have often struggled to find this balance in my clinical relationships with more provocative women. As Teresa and I started this second session, I was immediately feeling very anxious and confused.

Discussion Question: *What might be some of the cultural/gender-based implications of what was happening in these most recent interchanges in Theresa's therapy?*

____

____

____

Teresa started our session by telling me that she was upset with her boyfriend because he lived far away and did not make much of an effort to spend time with her and her infant daughter. She seemed very angry and spoke in a way that somehow seemed to demand that her boyfriend make himself more available.

I reflected back to her that all of this must be very hard for her: to love someone who was never there for her. This led Teresa to relax a little.

I then asked her if she had ever addressed this issue with her boyfriend directly. She sighed in despair and nodded affirmatively; answering that, when she brought this subject up with him, they would usually have an argument, which would result in him coming to see her even less. As Teresa was telling me this, she looked like she didn't know what to do and was feeling hopeless and confused. I remember feeling a sadness that I wished I could run away from.

This was a dynamic that came up regularly in the first three months of our work together: Teresa coming to sessions dressed provocatively, telling me about her problems with her boyfriend, and seeming to feel defeated and hopeless when I would gently encourage her to address her relational problems directly. I remember constantly feeling uncomfortable, confused, and overwhelmed.

Teresa also told me that she was having a hard time finding a job, was becoming less and less emotionally satisfied with her relationship with her boyfriend, and was feeling frustrated with her parents for being very dismissive and critical of her. She described her father as always high on marijuana and her mother as always miserably depressed or talking to herself. All of this seemed to make Teresa feel very lost and alone.

When I would sit and listen to her without interrupting, she tended to frantically jump from topic to topic in rapid succession and become progressively more overwhelmed and angry. In turn, this made me feel overwhelmed. Often, I would interrupt her lengthy disclosures and ask her questions or gently direct her towards assertive communication skills and other problem-solving strategies. In response, Teresa would usually sink further back into her chair and stare at me as if she was listening in order to be polite, though waiting for me to finish so that she could tell me more about her suffering. This led me to feel very defeated about, what I felt, was a strong likelihood that I was not helping her feel better or solve her problems.

Furthermore, Teresa only attended one or two out of every three or four of her therapy sessions. I remember feeling frustrated about this until I spoke with her doctor and former therapist in order to get their impressions of Teresa. The doctor and former therapist were frustrated with Teresa because she missed at least eight out of every 10 sessions with them. Thus, it is interesting that her fairly poor attendance in our sessions was actually an improvement.

Then, almost abruptly, Teresa stopped coming to her sessions' with me altogether. She uncharacteristically missed several weeks of therapy in a row without calling in ahead of time.

Discussion Question: *What might be your immediate-internal reaction if you were Teresa's therapist? As in, what would you attribute Teresa's therapeutic disengagement to?*

____

____

____

____

I wondered to myself if I had done something wrong. When I would call to find out what happened, she would usually tell me that she did not attend therapy because she was either busy with other affairs or was feeling physically ill.

Usually, I tried to empathize with Teresa's various struggles. However, as her absence from therapy prolonged, I was feeling progressively more frustrated with her with each passing week. Beneath my frustration, I felt rejected and abandoned. Somehow, I knew that I needed to very carefully hold on to this frustration and not let it out on Teresa. My concern was that, if I let my frustration out on her, I would become like all the other unsupportive others in her life. I hypothesized that I would need to be more patient and understanding if I wanted to have a deeper relationship with her. Meanwhile, I felt like I was trying to chase her back into therapy, though I sensed that this might ultimately be an opportunity to show her that I was worth taking an emotional chance on.

I decided to act on this premonition when the timing felt right. In one of our many phone conversations in between missed sessions, I asked Teresa how she felt about how her therapy was going.

She reported that she didn't feel like she was getting better and routinely spoke to her mother about the hopelessness of it all. She told me that her mother told her that she needed a therapist who was really willing to "go through it" with her; meaning someone who could help her open up emotionally and more deeply explore her inner life. Her mother seemed concerned that this would be emotionally difficult for the therapist as well. I reflected to myself that Teresa's mother was right.

Without thinking, I told Teresa that I would be willing to "go through it with her" if she was ready to let me. I heard her sigh on the other end of the phone.

Then, there was a long silence. I always wanted to know what she was thinking in those moments, but I felt obligated not to interrupt her. We then casually conversed for a couple more minutes before hanging up.

There-after, Teresa began to attend her sessions much more regularly and wore noticeably more clothing. I almost wanted to inquire about this, but elected not to because I couldn't think of any way to do this that wouldn't feel shaming.

Despite this more obvious physical change, the core emotionally-related themes in our therapeutic work remained largely the same. Teresa would often tell me about several of her life-problems in rapid succession, we would try to problem solve, we would fail to reach any real sense of resolution, and then we would both end up feeling anxious and overwhelmed.

In this middle phase of our work together, Teresa often expressed concern about her daughter's aggressive behavior at school, her father having lost his job and resigning himself to daily marijuana smoking on the couch, and her myriad of psycho-somatic pains and bodily symptoms. She seemed most worried about not knowing why she was having these bodily symptoms and was scared that they might be symptoms of Lupus; which she had learned about in high school.

In response, I would often educate her about the benefits of seeking medical care, diet, exercise, deep breathing, and relaxing uses of leisure time. I would also encourage her to come up with her own ideas about what she could do to physically and emotionally take care of herself outside of therapy. Teresa's face would then flatten and her eyes would fall to the floor or soften in a sad kind of way as she waited politely for me to finish speaking. Once I was finished, she would resume telling me that she was worried about her health, her daughter, and her father. This dynamic would usually lead Teresa to feel frantic and overwhelmed, which usually made me feel frantic and overwhelmed.

Discussion: *Describe one of your own clinical experiences of working with a client-of-color who seemed not to get better no matter what you did. Do you have any new insights into your case after reading about Teresa's therapy? If so, please describe.*

___

___

___

___

___

___

___

All the while, I felt like I was completely inadequate. When I listened supportively, she seemed to demand that I do something more. When I tried to gently direct her toward various problem solving strategies, she looked at me as if I might have done something wrong. I also remember feeling very anxious about an underlying sense of despair that was rapidly making its way to the surface. Whereas this type of anxiety would usually compel me to take corrective action, about nine months into my therapeutic work with Teresa, suddenly, finally, *I got it.*

"Teresa," I asked her. "Do you ever feel like nothing is ever going to get better and that that's really scary and so you have to keep trying different ways of fixing things but nothing works right and that makes you wanna' give up?"

"YEAH!" She fairly yelped, leaning forward in her chair, sitting up more rigidly, and staring hard at me as if she was both amazed and relieved. She then sat back, sunk even further back into her chair, and began to breathe more slowly and calmly. It felt to me like this might have been the first time that she ever really felt understood. I too couldn't help but to breathe a sigh of relief. That was a moment in our therapeutic work that seemed to last much longer. Somehow, after that, we were much, much emotionally closer.

Since then, in the last year or so of our therapeutic work, Teresa has rarely missed a session. She occasionally dresses more provocatively, but usually when the hot weather justifies wearing less clothes. In session, she also tends to stay focused on what she is *most* worried about rather than introducing one topic and then rapidly changing from one topic to the next. This tells me that, now, she may be more comfortable with me and might even be better able to use our relationship to help her regulate enough to process her experiences more coherently.

Nevertheless, Teresa has continued to struggle mightily in the recent present. She often tells me about experiencing odd bodily symptoms and what may be infections. These symptoms scare her immensely, though she reports having had so much contact with doctors and emergency rooms in the past that she is reluctant to seek medical care.

After talking about her health problems, she sometimes mentions her various traumas. The traumas she has mentioned include her having been a former gang member who had been shot at and gang raped, and having been abducted and then sexually abused when she was seven. She has only mentioned these traumas once or twice in her four years of therapy with me. After briefly mentioning these traumas, she usually changes the subject to something less vulnerable. This always leaves me with a flurry of questions that I want to ask her about what happened. However, I have always felt a strong urge to let Teresa move away from whatever subject she no longer wants to discuss; particularly those subjects that might make her feel vulnerable.

When Teresa brings up her traumas and then moves on to other subjects, she often talks about the casual, romantic relationships that she tends to seek when she feels less emotionally connected to her longtime boyfriend. She reports that these casual relationships tend to give her some of the validation that she doesn't get from her boyfriend.

After discussing her romantic relationships for between 10 and 20 minutes, she usually moves on to discuss other areas of her life that she feels distressed about; including her struggles with finding and maintaining employment. She is very sensitive to criticism and therefore struggles with taking direction from her supervisors. My sense is that Teresa often gets confused or distracted at work, which usually leads her supervisors to intervene, which

Teresa tends to interpret as criticism, which makes her feel overwhelmed. This combination of limitations makes it particularly difficult for Teresa to function in an employment setting.

Teresa reports that she is more capable of managing herself when she is working only part-time, though the income that she generates from working part-time is not enough to provide for herself and her daughter. Thus, she is most interested in finding part-time employment where she can sell marijuana. In order to sell marijuana at work, she has to be on the phone a lot at work and then also has to regularly go out in front of the business to meet her customers.

When Teresa finds employers who are willing to allow her to do this, they are most often older men who make sexual advances upon her. She says that the forbidden nature of these relationships with older (often married) men is somehow attractive, which often leads her to get sexually involved with them. After a relatively short period of time, she usually feels guilty about cheating on her boyfriend, grows sufficiently disinterested in the more casual relationship with the supervisor, and then wants the casual relationship to end. After telling the supervisor that she wants the sexual relationship to end, she always seems to get fired for something unrelated. Teresa interprets this chain of events as a symptom of the unfairness of "the male-dominated system," which makes it impossible for women to get ahead. This leads me to feel impatient and irritated; mainly, because Teresa has an Associate's degree in para-legal studies and may therefore be capable of finding more legitimate and viable employment.

Teresa has told me that being sexual makes her feel powerful and that this is the only way that she feels that she can have any real, executive authority in her life. She has told me that, usually, when she behaves in more sexually provocative ways, men do as she pleases. She says this with a sense of accomplishment, though she also seems to be masking underlying feelings of sadness about her romantic relationships not being emotionally deeper and more fulfilling.

Discussion Question: *Re-consider the information presented in the previous chapter on trauma. How might have Theresa's presentation in therapy been influenced by her various traumas? At this point in the case, how would you work with Teresa's traumas and what would you guess would be most helpful to her?*

____

____

____

____

____

____

In session, I have sometimes re-framed Teresa's sexual behavior in terms of how it is a survival strategy. For example, I might say that she is doing what she has always had to do in order to get by, which sometimes includes getting into less emotionally healthy relationships. In response, Teresa typically nods her head a little, looks down, relaxes momentarily, and then quickly resumes telling me about how unfair her life is.

She says that she tries to rely on her faith in god to help her work through her various struggles, but that her repeated life-failures make her feel overwhelmed and hopeless. When she feels this way, she tries to channel her energy into productive activities; including exploring continuing educational opportunities and taking emotional care of her family members. Despite the fundamentally healthy and responsible aspects of these behaviors, Teresa usually seems to gets more productively active in effort to distract herself from painful emotions. She is often too overwhelmed to effectively engage in these behaviors, which usually leads her to feel confused and irritated. Now that I think about it, it might be therapeutically productive for me to gently present this narrative of Teresa's behavior *to her* in session.

This last point leads me to reflect on how I spend a lot of time in clinical supervision trying to figure out how to help Teresa. These consultation sessions always leave me feeling hopeful about what I might say to her in future sessions. More specifically, my supervisor has often suggested that I ask Teresa about her early life, what she hopes to accomplish as a result of coming to therapy, if she really wants to change her life and, if she does want to change her life, *what she would be willing to do* in order to change her life. However, the overwhelming feelings that always seem to come up for me as soon as Teresa and I get started always seem to drown out my ability to remember helpful interventions.

This leads me up to our work today. I remain thoroughly unsure of the degree to which I have been helpful to Teresa, though I do tend to ask her about how she feels her therapy is going at least once every six months. When I ask her, I am usually thinking about whether another therapist might be a better match for her. I now suspect that she may pick up on the ensuing emotional distance because she usually responds to my inquiry by putting up a strong and pre-emptive protest. She says that she isn't always sure about whether her therapy is helping her and how it has helped her *if and when* it has been helpful. Either way, she doesn't want to start over with another therapist. She has elaborated that she thinks of me as a best friend and has told her family members this when they demand to know what is she doing in therapy and why she continues to suffer emotionally in spite of having met with me for four years.

I sometimes ask myself similar questions, which usually leads me to feel like I have failed Teresa. At some point thereafter, I reason that she would not have been my client for four years or refused to be transferred to another therapist if I was completely unhelpful to her. I then resolve myself to continue to do what is in my power to help her get better. Interestingly, there is a parallel between this last reflection of mine, one of the recurring emotional themes in our work, and how both *Teresa and I* (as individuals) try to adjust to stressful experiences and painful feelings outside of our sessions. In each of the aforementioned experiences, there is a sense of defeat and hopelessness, which leads to an impulse to problem solve, which tends to not be very effective, which leads to overwhelming anxiety.

Thus, it may be that I can relate to one of Teresa's core emotional experiences, and that the chaos I sometimes feel in our relationship may be representative of the chaos that Teresa feels inside of herself and tends to create in her external environments; *including in our relationship*. From a more diagnostic perspective, this would be considered *projection*; which Bateman et al. (2003) and Diamond et al. (2003) note to be a defense that borderlines use in order to achieve a (false) sense of control and safety. From a more relational, client-centered perspective, it may be that Teresa has succeeded in getting me to more deeply understand what it is sometimes like to be her. Ultimately, at the deepest level, this may have been what she wanted all along.

DISCUSSION

I will now discuss the re-curing themes in my therapeutic work with Teresa in terminology that is consistent with the theories I presented in the first half of the paper. Although my work with Teresa was largely intuitive, I will show that the core concepts of these theories are helpful guideposts for the development of this case. This linkage back to theory is important because, in my experience, working competently with more highly disordered borderlines (like Teresa) requires an ability to more deeply understand (i.e. conceptualize and theorize about) what has happened in the therapeutic work *and then use this information to guide future sessions*; which I will discuss in more detail later.

Teresa has behaved provocatively throughout our work together. It would be easy to label her as hyper sexualized, seductive, and poorly boundaried and to dismiss the possibility of deeper meanings of this behavior on the grounds that these are typical symptoms of borderline pathology. My experience has been that, when I think about Teresa in this more diagnostic way, I feel more comfortable, in control, *and emotionally distant* in our sessions. Now that I think about it, when I have been more emotionally distant from Teresa's deepest emotional experiences, my interventions have tended to be less effective.

I have found it more helpful to our therapeutic work to consider that behaving provocatively has been Teresa's most reliable strategy for *connecting with men*, which has been her primary attachment strategy throughout her whole life. Thinking about Teresa in this more relational way has helped to change my uncomfortable feelings to empathy and sadness about the way she must think of herself. This way of re-framing Teresa's provocative behavior coincides with the principles of the more relationally-oriented theories of borderline pathology.

My sense is that Teresa has internalized a belief that the only way she can get her needs met is through behaving provocatively; which is a cognitive distortion, though it is also consistent with her experiences. This makes me feel sad because I know that Teresa wants emotionally deeper and more satisfying relationships, though she typically behaves in ways that are unlikely to attract emotionally healthier relational partners. Furthermore, she tends to resist the skills-oriented and effective communication-oriented therapeutic interventions that might help her learn to behave more securely in relationships.

Throughout our therapeutic work, I have tended to take Teresa's disclosures literally and then respond to her on a more surface-pragmatic level. For example, when she came to her 2nd session in more provocative dress and told me that she felt unhappy about her relationship with her boyfriend, I inquired about whether she had addressed her concerns with him directly rather than encouraging her to explore the deeper meanings of her disclosures and behavior in-session.

My working hypothesis has been that a more present-day, real time focus on what *Teresa can do to positively affect her life* may reinforce that she is competent and capable of resolving her more immediate problems. For example, if her family members spoke to her in a critical way and she responded by utilizing effective communication skills, she might feel better about the interchange and therefore decrease the level of emotional-relational crisis in her life.

At the same time, I am also reflecting that the meta-message of Teresa's anxious flurries tends to be that she is scared and doesn't know what to do about the overwhelming nature of her struggles. When I have tried to help her problem solve, such as by educating her about self-care practices and interpersonal communication skills, she tends to emotionally recoil, wait politely until I am done talking, and then try harder to get me to understand what she is going through. When I have stayed emotionally closer to her experiences without leaning in the direction of trying to change them, she seems to feel understood/validated, which seems to help her regulate. This was particularly evident in the middle, more pivotal phase of our work together.

This last paragraph demonstrates that Teresa tended to respond more positively to interventions that coincided with the DBT principle of validation and tended to struggle with interventions that coincided with the DBT principles of building skills and changing behavior. This supports the contention I made in the beginning of my paper about how Teresa's case would illustrate my aforementioned dilemma of therapeutic approaches.

This also speaks to the points I made earlier about how borderlines may have a hard time with more confrontationally-oriented treatments. I interpret behavior-change as a lesser sense of therapeutic confrontation because trying to change the client's behavior inherently reinforces (i.e. judges) that they are doing something wrong and therefore challenges them to behave more functionally. I am also wondering if Teresa's more positive response to validating interventions (than skill-building interventions) might have larger implications for clinical work with borderlines, though further study would be needed in order to test this hypothesis.

I often find it difficult to validate Teresa and openly acknowledge how difficult it is for her to change her behavior. This is difficult *for me* because Teresa so often talks about herself as if she is a helpless victim; which tends to make me feel irritated. My reaction is informative because Teresa often describes her family members and other service providers as irritably pushing her to seek more gainful employment and to focus more on her daughter than on the men she is dating. I concur that these are laudable goals for Teresa, though I have also noticed that she tends to take such direction as criticism, which usually leads her to feel bad about herself and then seek out less emotionally healthy relationships in order to feel better.

Discussion Question: *Consider your own clinical experiences with clients-of-color. Write about an experience where you attempted to provide what you felt was necessary therapeutic direction that did not seem to be acceptable to the client. Hypothesize about why the client may have resisted your therapeutic direction. Consider cultural dynamics.*

____

____

____

____

____

Throughout my work with Teresa, I have tried to walk the fine line of helping her take charge of her life through improved self-care and increasing her interpersonal effectiveness, though also reflecting on our interchanges in order to make sure that my more directive efforts with her are clinically appropriate and not based on counter transference. Now that I think about it, when I have been more directive with Teresa, I have often felt irritated or impatient (i.e. less emotionally regulated). My hope is that this realization of what Linehan (1993b) calls a therapy interfering behavior will help me be more mindfully aware *of my reactions* to Teresa in our sessions in the future.

LIMITATIONS AND CRITIQUE

The primary limitation of this paper is that it may be a false dichotomy to imply that therapy is necessarily *either* validating or directive; as I have implied in my thesis statement. In fact, DBT integrates both principles into an evidenced-based approach. I will admit that one of the ways I mentally sort through complex psychotherapeutic processes is to compartmentalize the information. Although this mental strategy often helps me understand the interplay of complex and interrelated therapeutic concepts, this strategy also risks oversimplification.

It may be that I am attracted to the DBT approach to treating borderlines because its methodology coincides with my more compartmentalized way of thinking. This approach necessarily diagnoses borderlines' emotional realities as a cluster of symptoms and then recommends that they be educated about various skills and encouraged to apply certain skills to certain symptoms in order to facilitate emotional regulation. Nevertheless, my more intuitive approach to helping Teresa build skills seemed less helpful to her than when I validated her. I will now theorize about why this might have occurred.

Most often, Teresa has been overwhelmed by a flurry of competing emotions. My sense is that the intensity of her emotions makes it difficult for her to think clearly, which may make it difficult for her to learn new skills and then apply relevant skills to her problems. This leads me to hypothesize that borderlines might need sufficient reassurance, validation, and other expressions of radical acceptance from their therapists in order to *regulate enough to think clearly* and therefore be more receptive to skills-focused interventions. In that sense, it may be that the therapist needs to more actively help borderlines regulate until they are (at least temporarily) emotionally stable enough to learn skills that can help them regulate on their own. This way of thinking aligns with my previously discussed conceptualization of the borderline's therapist as necessarily being in a more guiding, parental role.

At the same time, it is important to mention that, although I have some training in DBT, I am not fully trained in Linehan's original model, nor am I presenting my work with Teresa as a perfect case example of this approach. My personal therapeutic style and some of the more clinically significant interchanges in my work with Teresa coincided with some of the core principles of DBT, though my contribution to these interchanges stemmed largely from my intuitions about Teresa's needs.

On that note, Teresa's lack of positive response to my efforts to help her build skills or change her behavior could have had less to do with the general efficacy of the interventions themselves and more to do with more subtle relational factors like my *therapeutic timing* and my *therapeutic delivery*; which Linehan (1993a) noted are very important to working effectively with borderlines. I do tend to present with a stronger personality and presence in the therapeutic room and have experienced strong counter transference reactions throughout my work with Teresa. Additionally, Teresa has an extensive history of being traumatized by men. Thus, it might be that she emotionally recoils in our sessions, not necessarily because she (like other borderlines) can't tolerate therapeutic direction or skills-building interventions, but because I have sometimes been directive with her based on counter transference. It may also be that she emotionally recoils when she feels invalidated by yet another man trying to control her. I will need to discuss this therapy interfering behavior more in *clinical consultation/supervision*, which Linehan (1993a; 1993b) describes as vitally necessary to working competently with borderlines.

This last paragraph reminds me that, as I was reading about the cognitively-oriented theories, I was concerned that they mentioned relatively little about the impact of trauma on human emotional and mental processes. Instead, they seemed focused on how people emotionally and mentally adjust to their traumas in ways that heighten their suffering. This strikes me as making light of the overwhelming nature of trauma and conceptualizing posttraumatic survival in a way that blames the victim for not thinking more clearly and adjusting more functionally in spite of trauma's necessarily damaging effects on key neurobiological processes (Weber et al., 2004).

This leads me to consider that much of Teresa's symptomology could be related to her extensive history of trauma. Teresa's behavior is consistent with posttraumatic: hyper arousal, avoidance, and recreation. For example, when Teresa pulls me into anxiety-driven cycles of panic and problem solving, she may be succeeding in re-creating her trauma. Additionally, she has tried move on from her traumas (i.e. avoid emotional pain that may be related to her traumas) through compulsive spiritual practices and getting into relationships that seem to bring her some sense of power or comfort. These behaviors distract her from painful feelings, though they eventually lead to additional problems and more severe emotional deregulation; which is consistent with the effects of posttraumatic symptomology (Kimmerling et al., 2002). This discussion of trauma is important because Zanarini et al. (1998) noted that there is a high level of co-occurrence between borderline personality disorder and posttraumatic stress disorder. Thus, another limitation of my work with Teresa is that I may have de-prioritized the significant extent to which she remains affected by her history of trauma; which is consistent with my aforementioned critique of the earlier cognitively-oriented theories.

As I now reflect back on the last four years of our work together, my sense is that Teresa has really wanted me to hear and understand her traumatic suffering. More than anything, she seems to not want to be alone and appreciates when I offer her a sense of togetherness. In session, I have asked her if this is true and she has readily agreed.

This last paragraph reminds me of Beck et al.'s (2004) aforementioned concerns about how the Dialectical Behavior Therapeutic approach doesn't help borderline clients feel better. It may be that the skills-focused part of the Dialectical Behavior Therapeutic approach can help borderlines development necessary life-skills, though the emphasis on building skills and changing behavior inherently limits how much their traumatic suffering can be heard. This may partially explain Teresa's lack of positive response to my efforts to help her change her behavior.

After having written this paper, my hope is that I will find a way to stay emotionally close to Teresa's experiences and validate her feelings, though also help her learn new and more effective relational skills. This way of working clinically speaks to Linehan's (1993b) recommendation that borderlines' need their therapists to provide them with significant empathy *and also gentle direction.* It may be that the best way I can help Teresa learn the self-acceptance and self-worth that will help her relate to others more effectively is for me *to relate to her in the same emotionally balanced, reassuring, regulated, and secure way that I hope that she will eventually learn to relate to others*. Ultimately, this may be the best way to help Teresa regulate in session and internalize the interpersonal skills that can help her function more effectively.

Chapter 5

TRANSFORMING TRAUMA THROUGH STRENGTHS*

INTRODUCTION

One of the guiding principles of strengths-based social work is to start where the client is at the time. In practice, this means that the clinician should flexibly respond to the needs of his or her client. This will help the clinician build a therapeutic relationship.

I found this way of practicing to be particularly effective with Jena, who was a client of mine when I worked at a crisis clinic. In her intake, she told me that she had been raped about a year before she came in for treatment. Since then, she often abused drugs and had sex with men she barely knew while under the influence. As she told me about this, she seemed angry at herself and confused. I remember thinking to myself that it might be particularly complicated for me, a male therapist, to try to help her work through these issues.

In order to build a relationship with her, I had to carefully and flexibly follow my intuitions about how I should adjust my approach to meet her needs. Sometimes, this meant being more active and directive with her. At other times, I needed to listen supportively and just be there.

Psychotherapy integration offers a theoretical framework for practicing this way. I will discuss this theory in more detail later, and then present Jena's case as an example of what integrating Ego Psychology and strengths-based social work looks like in practice. I have chosen these two theories because, when I was writing up her case, I found that my way of working with her was largely strengths-based. However, Ego Psychology helped me conceptualize her development, including her early life and traumatic experiences, and what happened in her therapy. When I found that an integration of these two models helped me explain what happened with Jena, I felt inspired to research them in more depth. Through this research, I found that the theory of *ego strength* in Ego Psychology and how *resilience* in strengths-based social work helped me explain how therapy helped Jena heal.

In the first half of my paper, I will explore the relationship of these two theories *in theory*. Then, in the second half of my paper, Jena's case will be presented as an example of what integration (of Ego Psychology and strengths-based social work) looks like in practice.

---

* A version of this chapter was also published in *The Journal of Theory Construction & Testing*, Volume 16 Number 1, Published by Tucker Publications. It has been expanded in an effort to encourage wider dissemination of research on the subject.

I wanted to explain what happened in Jena's therapy because of the impressive gains she made in a short period of time. She was already a very resilient person and so was naturally predisposed to a quick recovery. At the same time, I was impressed by her coming to therapy with concerns about regularly abusing drugs and engaging in promiscuous sex, and then achieving 30 days of abstinence from drugs and being in a relationship that she felt better about after eight weeks of therapy. It has been my experience that, although resilient clients tend to recover from crisis fairly quickly, Jena recovered much more quickly and to a greater degree. Initially, finding a theoretical explanation was difficult because I had no particular therapeutic model in mind when I worked with Jena and wasn't able to pinpoint exactly how therapy may have helped Jena until long after it was over.

I did not practice from any one particular model because my work with Jena occurred earlier in my career when I did not know the models well enough to practice from one or another. Sometimes, this lack of knowledge led me to feel anxious. Ironically, this lack of knowledge may have been helpful to the work with Jena. I expect that, if I had more working knowledge of the models at that stage in my career, I might have more rigidly ascribed to one model or another rather than flexibly responding to my intuitions about what Jena needed from me in the moment. These intuitions lead me to focus, primarily, on Jena's strength. When I present her case, I will show how my focusing on her strengths helped her build ego strength.

Ego Psychology

I will now present theories of the ego, starting with the Freudian schools. Sigmund Freud theorized that human development begins with conflict in the tripartite psyche, which includes the id, ego, and superego. The id is where instinctual drives for sex and aggression come from. Because it is not always appropriate to gratify these impulses, the superego morally represses them.

Ultimately, it is in the nature of the drives to be discharged (A. Freud, 1966). The ego allows the drives to be discharged in socially appropriate ways by negotiating compromises between the id and superego. These compromises are reached through the defenses (A. Freud, 1966).

Freud's analysis of the ego led to elaboration of the defense mechanisms by ego psychologists, including his daughter Anna Freud, Heinz Hartmann, and Erik Erikson. They founded Ego Psychology and made the ego their clinical center piece. They held on to the Freudian principle that the ego was a defensive structure, but added that the ego is inherently adaptive and has implications for human development (Mitchell et al., 1995). S. Freud was interested in how the defenses repressed reality. The ego psychologists were more interested in how people use their defenses to adapt to conflict, both in their psyches and *immediate-surrounding environments* (Mitchell et al., 1995). I say "immediate surrounding environment" because it was in the theory and practice of strengths-based social work that theories of the ego encompassed larger systemic issues. Ego Psychology considered the role of the environment in human development, but in a more narrow sense. It considered that development may be influenced by culture and experiences in the parent-child system, though intra psychic deficiencies were considered the most influential factors. Strengths-based social work went a step further by looking at the larger influence of society, and how psychic development may be influenced by oppression. This is one important way that strength based social work practice theory expanded upon Ego psychology's founding principles. This will be discussed in more detail later.

The Freudian defenses were regression, repression, reaction formation, isolation, undoing, projection, introjection, turning against the will, reversal, and sublimation, (Blanck et al., 1994; A. Freud, 1966, p. 44; Goldstein, 1984). I have listed them in order from least mature to most mature, as noted by A. Freud (1966). A. Freud noted that reaction formation is the individual's unconscious effort to hide his or her true feelings by behaving in the exact opposite way. A. Freud (1966) also noted that sublimation is the channeling of primitive feelings into productive activities. S. Freud noted that sublimation was the strategy by which the drives became adaptive (Mitchell et al., 1995). I have explained reaction formation and sublimation because those were Jena's most prominent defensive strategies. In the beginning of our work together, she more often used reaction formation. At the end of our work together, she had experiences that were consistent with sublimation. Though this is not meant to imply that we worked through her defenses in eight weeks, I will demonstrate that she may have used more mature defenses toward the end of our work together because her ego had grown stronger. I will also show how I helped her do this by helping her build resilience, which was one of her strengths to begin with. The underlying principle of Ego Psychology that supports my way of working with her is that the ego grows stronger when people use their internal resources to survive through and adjust to conflict.

This parallels Hartmann's (1958) theory of adaptation, which is one of the core principles of *Developmental Ego Psychology.* This school also included Spitz, Erikson, and Jacobson. They were among the first clinical theorists to look more deeply at infants' experiences in their surrounding environments. Margaret Mahler, for instance, developed a theory of separation and individuation. This theory was that young children are initially very dependent on their mothers and then gradually develop a more separate sense of self.

Hartmann pioneered a theoretical shift from a focus on intra-psychic structures and their dysfunctional effects to a focus on healthy and adaptive development. In contrast to others before him who saw ego development as dominated by conflict, Hartmann saw it as a progression. The ego develops along parallel tracks (personal communication, G. Bellows, 01/07/10). One is in conflict, the other in *conflict-free capacities within the id and ego.* These capacities include perception, memory, motor coordination, language, gifts, and talents (Hartmann, 1958). As long as there is, at least, *an average expectable environment,* these conflict-free capacities develop into ego functions and are able to function independently from the drives.

Like Hartmann, Erik Erikson formulated progressive theories of the ego. He expanded existing psychoanalytic theories of ego development into a psychosocial model which covered the whole lifespan. Erikson theorized that development happens organically through a series of growth crises or stages typified more by the concept of tension than conflict (Mitchell et al., 1994). His research led to the identification of eight interrelated psychosocial stages. These stages included trust v. mistrust, autonomy v. shame and doubt, initiative v. guilt, industry v. inferiority, identity v. role confusion, intimacy v. isolation, generativity v. stagnation, and ego integrity v. despair (Erikson, 1963).

Despite its strong ties to the earlier conflict-based theories, Ego Psychology was rapidly growing more focused on principles that tended to dovetail with strengths-based social work, including inborn ability, developmental potential, person-in-environment phenomena, and internal resources. Erikson was one of the developmental ego psychologists who led this movement. He went a step further than his predecessors by identifying that the individual had a core in the self *and* in the community (Mitchell et al., 1994).

Erikson and Hartmann were among the first clinical theorists to consider human development in terms of how it was influenced by broader forces in the environment. Erikson agreed with his fellow Freudian ego psychologists: that the individual is pushed by the drives. He added that the individual is *pulled by social institutions* and that society is essentially "an extension of the ego in its campaign to regulate the drives," (Mitchell et al., 1994, p. 143).

Markstrom is a contemporary ego psychologist who theorized that eight ego strengths corresponded to Erikson's eight psychosocial stages. She tested her conceptualization of Eriksonian theory in multiple research studies and achieved validity and reliability for its core principles, including that there is a relationship between ego strength and: psychosocial development, self-esteem, receiving social support, and resilience (Markstrom et al., 1999; Markstrom et al., 2001; Markstrom et al., 1997; Markstrom et al., 2007). In the next section, I will show that the relationship of these concepts is congruent with the strengths-based model of social work practice. When I present Jena's case, I will show that these concepts had implications for Jena's development and how therapy helped her heal.

Erikson's eight psychosocial stages correspond to Markstrom's eight ego strengths as follows (Markstrom et al., 2007; Markstrom et al., 2001): *Hope* (for the future) emerges in infancy from the psychosocial stage of trust and is learned from positive experiences with the primary caregiver. *Will* (i.e. free choice, awareness, and self-restraint) is associated with justice in parenting and emerges in early childhood from its stage of autonomy. *Purpose* (i.e. goals) emerges in early childhood from the stage of initiative. This ego strength allows the ego to invest one's will more productively in the pursuit of goals free of inhibition. *Competence* emerges in adolescence from the stage of industry. Failure to develop this strength results in psychosocial inferiority and a lack of productivity. *Fidelity* (i.e. loyalty and fairness) emerges in young adulthood from the stage of identity. *Love* emerges in young adulthood from the stage of intimacy. If this ego strength is not achieved, the individual develops a sense of isolation and exclusivity. *Care* (i.e. interest in future generations) emerges during adulthood from the stage of generativity. If this strength is not achieved, the individual develops a sense of stagnation. The final ego strength is *wisdom* (i.e. hope translating into faith). Wisdom emerges in late adulthood from its stage of integrity v. despair. G. Bellows (personal communication, 01/05/10) stated that *resilience* v. resignation has been identified as the ninth ego strength. These ego strengths consolidate into *ego integrity,* which is a sense of positivity about one's life. All of these eight specific ego strengths are meaningfully related to the kind of resilience that both ego psychology and the strengths based perspective in social work practice tend to emphasize in their theory and practice.

Eda Goldstein's (1984) discussion of defenses and coping skills is another example of how Ego Psychology and strengths-based social work theory complement one another. Goldstein is a social worker/professor at New York University who has written extensively on the role of ego psychology in social work practice. Her position is that defenses and coping skills co-exist. Coping skills are often preferable, but both coping skills and defenses are necessary for survival. They are similar in terms of how they are both employed by the individual in order to provide protection and facilitate survival in times of stress. However, they diverge markedly in terms of how they function.

Goldstein (1984) noted that defenses are rigid and automatic, whereas coping skills are flexible in the sense that the individual has more power to choose how and when to apply them. Defenses distort reality, while coping skills orient one's experience to reality. Coping involves a multiplicity of consciousness, while defenses try to repress consciousness. Goldstein's (1984) principles of positive coping within a multi-dimensional reality, and her view that people who are suffering should focus on the present and future rather than the past are consistent with the strengths-based model of social work practice.

Discussion Question: *Consider a recent experience you may have had with a client-of-color who was facing severe life challenges and was also difficult for you to therapeutically engage with. Was the client primarily using coping skills or defenses? Why might this be important to consider when meeting with this client for therapy?*

____

____

____

____

The Strengths-Based Model of Social Work Practice

When I first started my Masters of Social Work program, I was immediately drawn to this strengths based model. I was put off by clinical theories which seemed most interested in what people were doing wrong and how they were defective. The strengths-based model seemed to celebrate clients' impressive stories of survival.

Social work clients often present for therapy with multiple layers of problems, including living in dangerous neighborhoods, being oppressed throughout their lives, and being deprived of education and resources. Given that, it is understandable that clients would come to therapy with impairments in functioning. What is amazing is that social work clients come to therapy in as good shape as they do, despite the harshness of their surrounding environments. Strengths-based social work acknowledges that clients come to therapy with impairments in functioning, though these impairments are conceptualized in terms of systemic rather than psychic deficiencies (Saleeby, 2009).

Discussion Question: *How might the strengths-based principles of social work practice be helpful to facilitating therapeutic relationships with more severely suffering clients-of-color?*

____

____

____

____

According to the theory of strengths-based social work, it is the clinician's duty to help clients explore and re-claim the survival strategies and other internal resources that likely helped them survive through hard times in the past. Clients will experience such an approach as both validating and empowering, which will strengthen them internally so that they are better able to apply their internal resources to their external challenges (Saleeby, 2009).

A social work client's internal resources often consist of their natural talents and abilities, as well as their cultural, creative, and spiritual practices (Lum, 2003). Saleeby (2009) noted that, when social work clients present for therapy, these internal resources are still there, although the client may have forgotten about them due to the overwhelming nature of his or her presenting circumstances. If the client uses these internal resources to cope with and work through presenting challenges, he or she will grow internally stronger. This will better prepare the client for repeating this process as needed in the future (Benard, 2004). This is essentially Hartmann's theory of development applied to clinical practice, and is also a functional example of how *resilience* is built. When I present Jena's case, I will show what building resilience looks like in practice. Saleeby (2009) noted that resilience explains why most at-risk youth grow up to be fairly emotionally well-rounded adults. Markstrom et al. (1997) found that resilience was a key determinant of ego strength relative to the individual's corresponding psychosocial stage.

Early in my career, I liked the idea of a clinical relationship that was more egalitarian than hierarchical and sought to help clients help themselves. However, I struggled with this principle when I met with social work clients who interacted with me as if I was a doctor who was in a position to fix them. Though I strongly believed that a collaborative relationship would help my clients, I intuitively sensed that I needed to hold the position as an authority that they put me into. I found that being able to hold this position without encouraging it gave them the *hope* they needed to engage in and more actively participate in therapy.

Discussion Question: *What might be some of the cultural implications of therapist being related to as an authority figure? How might you use your inevitable position of power to empower the client?*

____

____

____

____

____

____

Saleeby (2009) noted that the primary purpose of strengths-based social work should be to inspire clients to be hopeful again. This is so important because it is the strength of the relationship that most often determines whether healing occurs. Saleeby (2009) noted that whether the relationship inspires the client to be hopeful is the strongest in-treatment predictor of positive clinical outcome. Similarly, the common theme in Markstrom's conceptualization of psychosocial theory was that developmentally appropriate internalized senses of competency and ability tended to be the markers for continuing psychosocial maturity.

My point about needing to hold the position the client put me into is an example of one of the key principles of strengths-based social work practice: that clinician's should seek to understand the client's cultural reality and respond in ways that coincide with the practices of that system (Lum, 2003). This is another way in which strengths-based social work takes the principles of Ego Psychology a step further. Erikson noted that cultural considerations have a relationship with psychosocial development. Strengths-based social work stresses that culture is not merely one factor among many that makes up the client's reality. Rather, a client's culture *is their reality* (Lum, 2003; Saleeby, 2009).

The primary principle of the clinical relationship in the strengths-based social work model of practice is that the clinician should be a collaborative supporter and hierarchy should be minimized (Wachtel et al., 1997). It will be better for the client to help him or herself heal, rather than for the healing to occur as a result of the benevolence of a superior clinician. Saleeby (2009) noted that such hierarchy is a reinforcement of the very oppression that may be contributing to the client's problems and keeping him or her from getting out of crisis. Similarly, Markstrom et al. (2001) concluded that an internal locus of control is more conducive to ego strength than an *external* locus of control.

Saleeby (2009) acknowledged that a power differential is inherent in any professional helping relationship. He advocates that clinicians should use their inevitable position of power to empower clients to make their own choices. For example, a client may tell a clinician about a family conflict and ask the clinician what to do. The clinician who seeks to empower the client could tell the client to do what he or she feels is right. Empowerment is defined by Wachtel et al. (1997) as the power to influence one's own life by making choices. This concept grew out of the Humanistic movement, particularly Rogerian theory. Empowerment is also one of the primary principles of the postmodern theories, which grew out of strengths-based social work, and include the Feminist, Solution-Focused, Social Justice, and Narrative Therapies.

This way of working with clients speaks to Wachtel's (1993) noted *strength-based therapeutic conversation*, in which therapy affirms and builds on client's strengths through confrontations or interpretations which are less threatening. For example, a clinician may tell a client who struggles with being open and expressive that he or she is *more open at some times than others.* This can gently push open the possibility for the client to move in the direction of deeper analysis.

Another advantage of the strengths-based social work model of practice is that clients often present with considerable damage as a result of oppression, and may lack the ego strength that is necessary to tolerate deep exploration. Goldstein (1984) theorized that when clients present in ways that suggest weak ego functioning, clinicians should be more active, supportive, and focused on the client's present day thinking and observable circumstances. According to Goldstein (1984), this more strengths-based way of practicing will help the client build ego strength. When I present Jena's case, I will show that I intuitively worked with Jena in this integrated way.

INTEGRATIVE PSYCHOTHERAPY

The core principle of integrative psychotherapeutic practice is that no one clinical theory is comprehensive enough to meet all of a client's needs (Wachtel et al., 1997). Client's needs are complex and ever-changing, thus it may be that any one particular model may be helpful at some times and not so helpful at other times. As each model has strengths and weaknesses, it does not make sense for clinicians to more rigidly subscribe to one model or another. Rather, clinicians should pull together the best interventions from many models so that the therapeutic work is more comprehensive. The decision about which model to use in which situation should be based on the clinician's professional experience, training, education, consultation with colleagues, relevant personal experience, and other use-of-self factors (Corey, 2009).

Though I didn't know it at the time that I was working with Jena, I was intuitively using the integrative method. Sometimes, I felt like I didn't know what I was doing because I wasn't following any one particular therapeutic model. When I present Jena's case, I will show that I flexibly adjusted my approach based on my intuitions about what she needed from me in the moment. Sometimes, she needed me to sit and listen. Sometimes, she needed me to challenge her. Sometimes, she needed me to interpret her behavior. It has been my professional experience that this complex array of presenting needs is typical of most highly traumatized social work clients. I will present my work with Jena as an example of how the integrative method can be effective in such instances.

Gurman et al. (2005) noted that there are four subtypes of integrative psychotherapeutic practice: Technical Eclecticism, Common Factors, Theoretical Integration, and Assimilative Integration. In technical eclectic practice, the clinician does not start with any one particular model. Instead, he or she may use two or more models depending on what the client needs in the moment. When the client's needs change, the clinician may change the approach. The clinician makes the decision about which model to use, primarily, based on his or her professional experience. When I present Jena's case, I will show that this was the subtype of integration that I intuitively used when I worked with her.

"Common factors" asserts that, if therapy is to help the client, certain *common factors* must be present, regardless of which therapeutic model the clinician may prefer (Gurman et al., 2005). These factors include: that a therapeutic alliance must be established, the clinician needs to be warm and have a positive regard for the client, and both the clinician and client must believe that treatment can provide the client with a corrective emotional experience.

In the Assimilative Integrative approach, the clinician starts with one particular model, but is willing to integrate other models in treatment as needed (Gurman et al, 2005). Assimilative Integration may be efficacious when one model helps the clinician think about a client, but adding additional models makes treatment more effective.

Theoretical Integration is the most complex and challenging of the four subtypes of integrative practice. This method is about trying to integrate the approaches of many different models in order to build a grand unified theory (Gurman et al., 2005). Similarly, Corey (2009) noted that, by combining the best elements from multiple models, more complete theoretical orientations can be developed and treatment can become more efficient. When I was writing this paper, I wondered about whether this was possible. When I found that ego strength and resilience were core principles of Ego Psychology and strengths-based social work, I felt more able to explain Jena's life and what happened in our work together.

JENA

I will now present Jena's case and conceptualize her therapy through the integration of ego psychology and the strengths-based theory of social work practice. I will describe what actually happened in her therapy in enough detail so that my reader can get a sense of what Jena was really like and what it was like to be in the room with her. This may help to establish a clinical basis for some of my less traditional interventions. In the first half of my paper, I introduced the basic principles and core theories that make ego strength and resilience applicable to practice. I will show that these concepts are applicable to practice by showing that I intuitively worked with Jena in a more strengths-based way that coincided with her cultural reality, and that this helped her develop ego strength. My main role in helping her do this was to more parentally guide her psychic exploration and modulate her affect. These are ego psychological concepts which I am presenting at this point in my paper because they best capture how the therapy contained Jena until her natural store of resilience could help her stabilize from her presenting crisis state.

Jena came to my drop-in University-based mental health clinic one day because she wanted pills for her stomach aches. I was randomly assigned to do her intake and preliminary assessment. As the triage nurse handed me her chart, I looked out in the lobby and called her name. Jena got up from her seat and followed me into an intake room without looking up at me. She was strikingly attractive, though she was also wearing baggy clothes and a black beanie hat pulled low over her face.

As we sat down in the intake room, Jena looked very uninterested and eager to get this visit over with. I asked her how we could help her, to which she responded that she had been having stomach aches and was struggling to concentrate on her school work. I listened supportively and inquired about her symptoms, including when they started and when they increased in severity.

She responded somewhat irritably, "it started a year ago when I got raped. I can't focus on my work. I can't pay attention in class. My stomach hurts like shit, and now."

Suddenly, I felt a rush of emotion that I still can't name as any one particular feeling. I remember only that it was intense and that I felt it right when Jena said she was raped.

"Oh my god I'm sorry that happened to you!" I blurted out: raw and genuine. Jena looked up slightly from the floor to a meaningless spot on the wall, as if she just now recognized that I was in the room with her. She began to cry and went into a long, emotionally charged, and complex narrative that tended to chaotically jump around from one time in her life to another.

First, she told me about the young man at her school who got high with her at a party, and then fairly invited himself back to her dorm room with her. After he violently raped her, the police showed up and interviewed her in a way that made her feel like she was the perpetrator. "You invited him to your room? You didn't yell out? Mmm-hmm," the responding male officers inquired of her. As she told me this story, Jena tended to go back and forth from crying quietly, to staring hard at me while she angrily condemned her assailant and the interviewing police officers, to crying quietly again.

After a half an hour of this, Jena looked up at me and seemed suddenly more aware that I was listening closely to her with a concerned look on my face. She sat straight up in her chair and stared hard at me as if she might throw a punch. I felt frightened and small and wondered what I had done to make her so angry. It may have been that Jena became aware that she was presenting as vulnerable and responded by asserting her ability to protect herself, which would be consistent with the defense reaction formation.

Jena went on to tell me that she used to be in a gang and often engaged in violent behavior, including robbing a casino and being shot at several times. She proudly informed me that being in a gang provided her and other poor young Latinos/as in her neighborhood with an opportunity to: "be a somebody in a place of nobodies."

Discussion Question: *What values would Jena probably have learned from being in a gang? How might those values manifest during her recovery from being raped? As in, how might her core values make it particularly challenging for her to recover, and what are your thoughts about how to work with this in therapy?*

____

____

____

____

____

My sense is that Jena probably had to fight twice as hard to prove herself as a girl in a gang, and internalized a socio-culturally appropriate value for aggression and to despise anything reminiscent of weakness. I sensed that this mentality probably helped her survive in the projects, though it may have made it doubly hard for her to face the fact that she was raped. I could tell that she was trying to move on with her life as if the rape never happened, which may have been why she had such intense stomach aches. It may have been that she tried to repress the experience of being raped and then expressed her emotional pain in psycho-somatic symptoms. This demonstrates that Jena's survival skills were either ego-syntonic or ego-dystonic depending on what was happening in her surrounding environment. This supports my position on how strengths-based social work's broadening of the scope of the environment adds a clinically significant dimension to the ego psychological theory of adaptation.

Discussion Question: *Think back to the case of Theresa. Discuss any new ideas about her various challenges and any new hypotheses' you might have about how she presented in therapy and why.*

____

____

____

____

Throughout Jena's first session, I would listen supportively to her and non-verbally communicate to her that I understood her experiences and point of view. This coincides with the client-centered principles of strengths-based social work practice and the ego psychological principle of validation. When I would listen supportively, Jena would go deeper into her experiences. After a few minutes of this, Jena would grow very angry at herself for "letting *it* happen" and would de-regulate in a way that felt like she was overwhelming or re-traumatizing herself. This suggests to me that Jena's ego was weakened, possibly because it was damaged by her trauma. If her ego was strong and functional, she would be better able to process her experiences in doses that she could handle. If her ego was strong and functional and she started to feel emotional discomfort, she might change the subject or otherwise manage herself in a way that kept her regulated. Jena's tendency to decompensate when she explored her feelings suggests that her ego was not strong enough, at least in the face of the affect associated with her trauma, to initiate coping, which would normally help her remain regulated. She needed me to more actively guide her psychic exploration in a way that is consistent with the role of the analyst in classical ego psychology and A. Freud's (1966) theory of how parents need to guide their children's development in order for them to experience the adaptive successes that will help them grow internally stronger.

For example, when Jena de-compensated in session, I would normally step in and stop her by asking questions that encouraged her to consider a less punishing view of herself. This is consistent with Goldstein's (1984) theories of how to build the ego through cognitive therapeutic work. I would do this with Jena in a more actively assertive way, which tended to help Jena calm down rather than decompensating further. This positive response suggests that I was helping Jena modulate her affect as well as providing her with boundaries so that she could remain contained while she explored herself. This parallels A. Freud's (1966) theory of how parents serve as their children's auxiliary egos. Parents guide their children's development by providing them with validation and boundaries until their egos reach a more functional level of independence, which would be evidenced by a child being able to set and maintain boundaries on his or her own. Later, I will show that this theory supports that Jena's ego was stronger by the end of her therapy. My sense is that Jena may have been receptive to my efforts to help her because I was relating to her in a stronger, more assertive way that was familiar to her in her gang experiences. This is particularly important because more hardened clients like Jena are often less receptive to professional helping efforts.

In the first half of her first session with me, Jena went through a cycle of experiencing intense anger and then intermittent periods of regulation. After this cycle repeated a few times, Jena went on to resentfully tell me about how her mother used to beat her until she was old enough to carry weapons and defend herself. She told me that her mother's abuse reinforced her devotion to the gang because the gang accepted her and gave her a sense of purpose which she did not experience at home. In that sense, joining the gang was adaptive, or at least suggestive of the ego strength adaptive regression-in-service of the ego. Jena had to participate in violence in order to remain an active gang member, which might normally suggest that she made poor decisions concerning her welfare, which would normally suggest weak ego functioning. However, she described her gang involvement as a socio-culturally appropriate way for her and others like her to obtain validation and protection from would-be predatory criminals in her projects. Jena's experience was that she had to participate in violence in order to maintain what was essentially an auxiliary source of validation and boundaries. It is debatable that Jena joining a gang was adaptive, though it was important for our relationship that I understand her reality as she experienced it and not judge it. This supports Goldstein's (1984) recommendation that it may be helpful to incorporate strengths into an assessment of ego functioning.

After telling me about how her mother abused her, Jena went on to tell me that she was frustrated with herself because her grades were declining. She said that she used to be a straight-A student and was very dissatisfied with the B's and C's she had been receiving over this last year. She also told me that, once she was accepted to college, she promptly left the gang and that school had always been "her way out." This tells me that Jena was very resilient, particularly because her maintaining good grades shows that she was able to plan for the long term and delay gratification. These abilities are consistent with the ego strengths noted by Bellak, Hurvich, and Gediman (1973), the cognitive capacities that Goldstein (1984) noted suggest ego strength, and Markstrom et al.'s (1997) noted indicators of psychosocial maturity.

Discussion Question: *Did you expect Jena to be a stellar student? Why or why not? Is there a lesson to be learned from this?*

____

____

____

____

____

____

After Jena told me about her declining grades, I non-verbally communicated an understanding of why getting good grades was so important to her. Then, she started to talk about herself in a more harshly judgmental manner. She looked away from me and sat back in her chair as she told me that she was frustrated with her inability to study hard regardless of having unbearable stomach aches. At first, I gently questioned her harsh views of herself. She responded by more angrily asserting that she was stupid and lazy. This is consistent with Schiller's (2009) theories that a trauma survivor's superego may be punishing and that the survivor will look upon her victim-self with revulsion. When her self-deprecation became sufficiently intense, I felt that I needed to step in and more assertively protect her from herself.

"Jena, stop beating up on yourself!" I fairly demanded. For the first time in this first session, Jena stopped abruptly and looked like she might be more deeply reflecting on what she had just been saying. After a couple seconds of what felt like a productive silence, she laughed and endearingly called me her thug doctor.

I smiled shyly and looked up to see that two hours had gone by. I felt tired, but a little relieved. Jena seemed to be feeling the same way; it was as if we were both relieved that we had survived. I asked her if she might be interested in coming back again and she readily agreed. I was excited to think that our work could help her, though I doubted my therapeutic abilities; I had very little experience working with sexual trauma survivors and was also a bit overwhelmed by the complexity of her history.

I looked up at her in wonder and asked: "How can I help you from here? What should I do?"

She looked hard at me, as if both daring me to give her what she was asking for and doubting that I would: "Tell me straight up what's going on! I can take it!" This may support that she was engaging in M. Coombs' (personal communication, 06/10/09) stated tendency for clients to test their therapists in order to build mastery-competence capacities.

When I asked Jena if she was sure about wanting me to work with her in this way, she laughed from her belly; probably at my thought that she, a hardened gang member, might not be able to withstand a more challenging therapy. She seemed certain that this would help her and I felt obliged to respect her wishes. I remember considering that my agency permitted a maximum of only eight crisis-focused sessions, which gave me the sense that getting right to the point might be a good way for us to clinically make the most of our limited time together.

I was encouraged to see that, in the next few sessions of our work, Jena told me more about her present day issues than her past traumas, which is evidence that she was beginning to stabilize. This also supports Goldstein's (1984) theory that trauma may damage the ego, but that a survivor with a good showing of ego strength in the past may recover quickly.

In the latter half of her therapy, Jena still tended to beat up on herself for not being able to study for long periods of time without taking breaks. However, she did this without as much intense anger. She would also pause periodically in a way that gave me more opportunities to intervene and modulate her affect. My sense is that Jena still lacked the ego strength to regulate on her own, but that our relationship was deepening and she was beginning to trust me and feel safe in the therapy. This helped her become progressively more able to use my support to regulate. This suggests that her ego was stronger than when she began the therapy because she was developing an object relationship with me. Goldstein (1984) noted that object relations is often considered *the ego strength* which all other ego strengths tie into.

Later in her therapy, when she judged herself in this relatively less harsh way for her struggles with schoolwork, I would usually let her talk freely until she began to speak more loudly or with more pressure.

Discussion Question: *If you were Jena's therapist, at this point in the therapy, what might be some ways that you might attempt to help her modulate her affect? Consider her core cultural values and her trauma history so that you come up with interventions that she is likely to be able to therapeutically accept and tolerate.*

____

____

____

____

____

____

____

When this reached the level of feeling relentless and punishing, I would often interrupt her and inquire about whether she could take a break when studying. Then, maybe she could get back to her work after eating or taking a walk, which she mentioned were two of her primary coping skills. In this last half of her therapeutic work, Jena was less defensive and more amenable to coping. She never openly agreed to my suggestions, but would usually calm down in response. My sense is that I helped her by providing a container for her exploration, which I gradually widened as she seemed capable of safely going further. This is consistent with: A. Freud's (1966) theory of how parents help children build remedial ego strength by gradually allowing them to progress into developmentally-appropriate levels of independence, Markstrom et al.'s (1997) theory that parents help children progress into age-appropriate levels of psychosocial maturation, and Wachtel's (1993) noted strategy for how the therapist can go from his or her inevitable position of power to empowering the client.

In our last few sessions, when I would step in and interrupt Jena when she judged herself, she would often stop and more calmly look away into nothing. Then, she would sometimes tell me more about the rape. When she talked about the rape in the beginning of our work, she tended to express anger. When she talked about the rape in the last few sessions of our work, she more often shared her feelings of remorse that it happened. She would also *wonder* about whether she could have done something, but in a way that gave us much more room to explore the possibility that, maybe, she couldn't have done anything. This is consistent with Mui's (2005) theories about how to help female survivors recover from rape trauma. My sense is that the earlier stages of Jena's therapy helped her establish that she could be safe in the therapy, which helped her eventually explore her deeper, most painful feelings of loss and sadness with me. In these periods, I would often listen supportively and then gently encourage her to consider that women who have been raped often feel similar to how she felt. Smith (2003) noted that connecting a female rape survivor's experience to a larger issue can be a particularly powerful intervention, which I consistently emphasized toward the end of our work together. I repeatedly used this intervention when Jena experienced states of sadness and vulnerability in the hope that she might link her most deeply loathed feelings to a female-centric identity that was more ego-syntonic than her previous ego-identity of a helpless victim; the ultimate insult in her gang subculture. Markstrom et al. (1997) noted that, when clients develop more ego syntonic-identities, their egos will grow stronger and more capable of initiating functional adaptive processes. I intuitively sensed that Jena could not tolerate anything too feminine, but that survivorship might be strong enough for her to tolerate and feminine enough to help her have some empathy for herself.

My sense was that, when Jena felt painful feelings, her usual way of dealing with them was to defensively try and understand what was happening, which led her to judge herself harshly. I did not have enough time to try to change her defensive patterns, though it was possible that the therapy could help her think in more helpful ways. This therapeutic goal is consistent with the strengths-based principle of helping clients re-call and make use of the survival strategies that helped them survive through harsh circumstances in the past, which may be able to help them survive in the present. Benard (2004) noted that, when this occurs successfully, it will help clients build resilience, which was one of Jena's strengths to begin with. My hope was that, if I consistently linked Jena's deepest, most intolerable feelings to her being an oppressed woman, she might go right to this more empathic frame of reference when she felt painful feelings outside of therapy and that this might even prevent her from regressing back into a crisis state.

Jena often seemed dubious about my view of her as an oppressed woman. Nevertheless, in our last session, she came in and proudly informed me that she was presenting a piece of artwork that she made in an art show which showcased the work of female rape survivors. She also told me that she was determined to try to "help other women relate to each other". This is consistent with the strengths-based theory of empowerment, and Mitchell et al.'s (1995) definition of the defense sublimation.

Jena also informed me that she had been sober for thirty days and had stopped having sex under the influence of drugs with men she randomly met at parties. She went on to say that she had met a young man at school three weeks ago, and had been seeing him and only him ever since. She told me that she felt good about having let him know that they would not be having sex "for a long time". It may have been that, from a having a supportive relationship with me, she learned how to selectively trust men again and how to be in boundaried relationships with us. Thus, it may have been that my more active assertion of boundaries in our relationship modeled for Jena how to set and maintain firmer boundaries in her new relationship, which is consistent with A. Freud's (1966) theories about how parents help children develop functionally independent egos.

In summary, Jena was a very resilient individual, which helped her recover fairly quickly. She was also prescribed psychiatric medications in my clinic, which may have helped her feel some relief. My role in helping her stabilize was to modulate her affect while her medications and natural store of resilience helped her grow stronger. Modulating Jena's affect was a complex process because she was not the kind of client who would normally be very receptive to more traditional efforts to establish an empathic connection. As an example, when I would listen supportively to Jena or reflect the emotional content of her experiences back to her, she would tell me more about her experiences and then quickly de-compensate. This demonstrates that, while my empathy helped her feel safe enough to explore herself, she could not use it to regulate. Jena needed to explore herself so as to get out some of the painful emotions that would otherwise continue to be expressed psycho-somatically. However, she also needed to explore herself safely, which required that I more actively contain her. My willingness to do this in the stronger and more assertive way that she asked for was validating in and of itself, which may have helped Jena be more receptive to my interventions so that she could use them to emotionally self-regulate. This is an example of how the client-centered principles of strengths-based social work may help to get a traumatized client talking, but that it may be necessary to integrate the more parental aspects of ego psychology so that the client is both validated and contained. This all is particularly noteworthy considering that Jena only came to my clinic because she wanted to get pills for her stomach aches.

Critique and Conclusion

In this last section, I will summarize how the integration of ego psychology and strengths-based social work has been helpful in this case, what its strengths and weaknesses are, and what implications this research has for future practice. I will also answer some of these critiques in a way that shows what implications this exploration has for future practice.

The client-centered principles of strengths-based social work helped me work effectively with Jena. However, I found that the strengths-based perspective failed to account for the extent of Jena's psychological distress and overemphasized the resilience aspect of her functioning. Ego psychology partially helped me close this gap by providing a more developmentally-focused explanation of what happened in her therapy. However, neither model explained Jena and my emotional connection in the way that attachment theory would.

The main benefit of integrating strengths-based social work and ego psychology in Jena's case was that this integration helped me explain Jena's development in experience-near terms. This is important because Jena needed psychotherapeutic intervention to help her become more aware of her feelings, to work through her psychosomatic symptoms, and to face the reality that she was raped and work through the emotions related to the trauma in a way that helped her grow. However, the intervention needed to be in a form that she would accept. I found that Jena was receptive to my interventions because our work coincided with her cultural reality, a point that is virtually ignored in early ego psychology and is one of the core principles of the strengths-based model of social work practice.

Two of the most glaring limitations of my work with Jena was that she was paired with a male therapist and had only eight sessions of therapy. It may have been a beneficial match for Jena to be paired with a female therapist who could be a positive female role model for her. At the conclusion of our work together, she did in fact link to a female nurse practitioner at an outpatient women's clinic. Jena described this woman as being warm and kind in a way that was both hard for her to tolerate and, probably, what she needed the most. Jena said that, in their first meeting, the nurse practitioner listened supportively and was very gentle with her. Jena resentfully told me that this was the type of woman who she would have beaten up in high school.

Discussion Question: *Why might Jena have reacted in the way described to the gentle female nurse practitioner? What might be some of the deeper, clinical meanings of her reactions? Consider her cultural values.*

____

____

____

____

____

____

____

Ego psychology and strengths-based social work would view her reaction very differently. Analytically-focused ego psychology would view Jena as reacting strongly to the most loathed victim part of herself that this kind, gentle woman reminded her of. An analyst might see this as the perfect opportunity for Jena to work through a particularly meaningful transference. My concern is that this is a very pathological way to look at Jena, which would have guided the therapy in a way that she was unlikely to accept. The strengths-based perspective would consider that Jena was strong and assertive because this is what helped her survive in the projects. Furthermore, she didn't stay in therapy with me because she wanted to become soft and gentle in the way that early ego psychology would assume. Jena wanted to get back to her old, tough and resilient self. My role in helping her do this was to guide her development in a way that she would respond to.

A concern about this strengths-based way of working with her is that it makes light of the overwhelming nature of her presenting circumstances and may short change a deeper consideration of how her personality factors may have influenced the therapy. Similarly, my own overly active and encouraging mannerisms may have sent Jena the message that I expected her to get better. Thus it is possible that she only presented as more stable because this is what I wanted. This would coincide with the report of the Institute for Safe Medication Practice (2014): that Latinos/as often see the therapist as a doctor who must be deferred to out of respect for the position as an authority figure.

Another limitation is that we only had eight sessions to work together. Though I do believe that this time limitation helped us get right to work and was conducive to my own therapeutic style, there are obvious concerns about a male clinician being so directive with a woman who had been raped. Working with her in this way risked re-traumatizing her, which is why I closely monitored how she responded to my interventions. My sense was that, when I intervened more actively, she was able to calm down and refocus. Nevertheless, my being a white male inherently limits my ability to understand Jena's reality as a Puerto Rican woman.

My conclusion is that the integration of ego psychology and strengths-based social work offers a framework for connecting with highly traumatized social work clients, intervening in ways that support healthy development, and explaining what happens in therapy in ways that account for inter-psychic conflict and environmental phenomena. This supports Corey's (2009) point about how no one therapeutic model has all the answers, though integrating the best points from multiple models allows clinician's to connect with clients on all levels of human experience

Chapter 6

Traversing Two Worlds: Family Therapy with an East Indian Adolescent Substance Abuser*

Introduction

East Indians are one of the fastest growing immigrant groups in the United States that has a population of over one million (Baptiste, 2005). As of 2005, India was the country that had the 3rd highest rate of immigration to the United States (Baptiste, 2005). The 2000 census reported that the East Indian population in the United States was 1.5 million, was growing at an average rate of 7.6% annually, and made up 0.6% of the total U.S. population and 16.4% of the Asian-American population (Poulsen, 2009). In the 2000 – 2001 academic year, East Indians made up 10% of the international student body in the United States (Poulsen, 2009). It is therefore increasingly likely that many American therapists will treat an East Indian immigrant family at some point in their careers, which underscores the need for further study on this topic (Baptiste, 2005).

I decided to write this paper after recently doing family therapy with the East Indian family of a 14 year old adolescent female who was involuntarily hospitalized due to alcohol-induced psychosis. Her family of five immigrated to the United States from the smaller East Indian region of Bangalore 18 months prior to initiating family therapy at the insistence of the local emergency room. Referent hospital staff informed me that the family experienced significant inter-familial conflicts since immigrating to America, which 14-year-old *Sanjita* may have been abusing alcohol to cope with.

I decided on a traditional family therapeutic approach given my training in traditional family therapy and my experience that a traditional therapeutic approach is often an effective treatment for adolescent substance abuse (Shelef et al., 2005). I also found myself needing to flexibly adjust my therapeutic approach based on my sense of the families' needs, which is consistent with recommendations from research on family therapy with East Indians (Poulsen, 2009; Baptiste, 2005). Sometimes, I needed to meet with all family members and focus

---

* With kind permission from Springer Science + Business Media: A version of this chapter was also published in *Contemporary Family Therapy*, Volume 35(4), 2013, published by Springer. It has been expanded in an effort to encourage wider dissemination of research on the subject.

exclusively on substance abuse. Sometimes, I needed to work with individual family members (mainly the father) on communication skills and parenting practices.

The most encouraging result from this case was that Sanjita's father decreased *his own substance abuse* and improved his parenting practices, which lead to decreased family conflict, the primary risk factor for Sanjita's alcohol abuse. The father's improvements are particularly noteworthy because research on East Indian immigrant families implies that the fathers' typically domineering and authoritarian role in the home is virtually impenetrable and clashes with their adolescents' fairly rapid acceptance of American cultural values (Baptiste, 2005). My case demonstrates that decreasing parental substance abuse has potential to improve family functioning, even when those improvements seem to be in contrast with traditional East Indian cultural values.

Positive therapeutic outcomes inspired me to write up this case and attempt to explain what happened and why through clinical theory. Through research and reflection, I concluded that my therapeutic approach to Sanjita's family mostly aligned with the principles of *multi-dimensional family therapy* (MDFT), a traditional family therapeutic approach to adolescent substance abuse treatment that has consistently achieved noteworthy results (Liddle et al., 2009; Henderson et al., 2010). Research also supports that traditional family therapeutic approaches are effective with East Indian families because traditional family therapeutic principles are consistent with traditional East Indian cultural values, which I will explain in more detail later (Baptiste, 2005). My case will corroborate the logical next step of these two findings by providing preliminary support for a multi-dimensional family therapeutic approach *to East Indian adolescent substance abuse and parent-child relational problems*.

In this paper, I will first present a history of East Indian immigration, some literature on East Indian cultural and family values, and a brief overview of the core operating principles of the multi-dimensional family therapeutic approach to adolescent substance abuse treatment so as to establish a context for my case. I will then present the case and use relevant research on East Indians' and MDFT to support my most clinically significant interventions, conceptualizations, and hypotheses'. I will show that the family members, particularly the father, tended to accept and respond most favorably to my interventions that coincided with the principles of traditional East Indian culture and MDFT.

EAST INDIAN IMMIGRATION TO THE U.S.

East Indians have immigrated to the United States since the late 1800's/early 1900's (Baptiste, 2005; Poulsen, 2009). East Indian immigration occurred, primarily, in two distinct periods – the early 20th century to 1924 and 1965 to the present (Baptiste, 2005).

The first wave of Indian immigrants to the US was mostly poor Sikh farmers from the Northern Indian state of Punjab who settled in California in search of work as loggers and railroad workers (Baptiste, 2005; Poulsen, 2009). A minority of these first-wave immigrants were middle-class businessmen, skilled craftsmen, and educated professionals (Baptiste, 2005; Poulsen, 2009). Immigration was considered a temporary maneuver by men who left their families in India in the care of their extended families until they could return to India with earnings (Poulsen, 2009).

The second period of immigration took place after the U.S Immigration and Naturalization Act of 1965 (Poulsen, 2009). This legislation emphasized family reunification, though attempted to restrict East Indian immigration to those that were highly educated, English speaking, and financially stable (Poulsen, 2009). This second wave of immigration included a mix of farmers, skilled and unskilled workers, and highly educated professionals such as doctors, physicians, and academics (Baptiste, 2005).

East Indian men who immigrate to America in contemporary times continue to support aging parents and their extended families through sending money and other resources back to India, even while they continue to establish their careers and home life in America (Poulsen, 2009). East Indian immigrants also help each other through assisted sponsorship, providing emotional support, and sharing resources with newly immigrated family members (Poulsen, 2009).

East Indians often immigrate to the United States to escape dismal economic and social conditions (Baptiste, 2005). East Indian families in India are often organized in "joint families," which may involve up to three or four generations of families living in one house with each family living together in their own separate room (Medora et al., 2003). Joint families share household responsibilities, including child and elderly care, running errands, social entertainment, income, and common property areas, and cook meals under one hearth (Medora et al., 2003). The author notes that East Indians in America often continue to organize themselves in joint families. Although this suggests obvious familial and cultural strengths, it also speaks to the extreme poverty of East India and explains why East Indians immigrate to America to improve their education, professional opportunities, and economic status, and to otherwise pursue a better life for themselves and for their families (Medora et al., 2003; Baptiste, 2005). This proscribed trajectory towards education and professionalism helps Indian families stabilize in the aftermath of immigration (Poulsen, 2009).

Like other Asian minorities, East Indians' strong familial connection and relatively healthy psychological adjustment to U.S. culture lead them be considered among the *model minorities* although, outside of employment and education, they often only associate with other East Indians and create what Poulsen (2009) calls *mini-Indias in America*. In spite of being a fairly well-adjusted immigrant group, East Indian families are often ambivalent about moving the United States due to fundamental disagreement with the core US cultural values, including what they learn from television, news reports, or from relatives already in the U.S.; particularly about child-rearing practices, which I will discuss in more detail later (Baptiste, 2005). East Indian immigrant families often maintain a social distance from US culture so as to retain their native values, ideologies, and beliefs, which may vary significantly depending on exactly where in Southeast Asia they are from and may also lead to cultural clashes which can make adjustment to U.S. culture increasingly difficult (Baptiste, 2005; Poulsen, 2009; Kwak et al., 2001). This common struggle of East Indian immigrants will be shown to have implications for my case.

EAST INDIAN CULTURAL VALUES

I will first discuss traditional East Indian values and then illustrate how they guide East Indian family structure, parenting practices, and gender-role conformity *in India and*

America. I will show that these cultural values provide East Indian's with a sense of *group identity* and connection, albeit at the cost of individual identity development, particularly for women (Medora et al., 2003); a dichotomy which will be shown to have implications for Sanjita's families' conflict.

Most East Indian immigrant families are Hindu and tend to maintain traditional Hindu values for interdependence, tolerance, diversion, conformity, harmony, and a stronger sense of connection to the family and the larger East Indian community (Medora et al., 2003; Dattilio et al., 2005; Baptiste, 2005). Traditions that are practiced faithfully include speaking the native language in the home, cooking Indian food, following religious and cultural customs, and caring for elderly parents (Poulsen, 2009). Most East Indian families devote a small portion of their private homes to a small Hindu shrine, Sikh prayer room, or some other designated area for prayer and meditation (Poulsen, 2009). This helps to create a sense of community and ongoing connection to traditions, values, and the spiritual life of India (Poulsen, 2009).

This faithfulness to traditions remains strong regardless of level of acculturation to U.S. culture, is a source of support and cultural and ethnic identity, permeates daily life, and is reinforced by parents for the betterment of younger generations (Poulsen, 2009). This demonstrates that East Indians have both a past *and future* orientation that brings a social obligation to ones' family and community (Poulsen, 2009). Actions in the present have ramifications for the reputation of both past and future generations, which is a cultural value that stems from religious and philosophical beliefs that emphasize ethical behavior, transcendental values, and self-actualization (Poulsen, 2009).

Discussion Question: *Given traditional East Indian cultural values, what would you imagine are the primary challenges facing East Indian families immigrating to the United States? How might you orient therapy so that it coincides with traditional East Indian values ?*

____

____

____

____

____

THE TRADITIONAL EAST INDIAN FAMILY

"The family in India has served as the basic unit of human social life," (Medora et al., 2003, p. 418). Family is treasured and is seen as a necessary part of the life cycle (Dattilio et al., 2005). East Indians families are generally strong, resilient, enduring, and well-structured, and have been throughout history (Medora et al., 2003). Family members are generally close, mutually interested and connected, bonded for life with relatives, and influenced by strong interfamilial-group controls (Medora et al., 2003). The extended family and "fictive kin" also play a very important role in the East Indian family and have maintained this important role despite the significant impact of urbanization and industrialization (Natarajan et al., 2005; Medora et al., 2003).

East Indian families are traditionally patriarchal and hierarchal in a way that mirrors the authoritarian nature of primary institutions in India (Garg et al., 2005). The father is the undisputed head-of-household and primary decision-maker, which he is prepared for through being raised in childhood to be less tolerant, independent, assertive, self-reliant, demanding, domineering, and heavily invested in his career and hobbies (Medora et al., 2003). Regardless of education or employment skills, men are expected to work outside of the home and financially support their families (Baptiste, 2005).

The East Indian mother is usually wed to the husband through a marriage that is arranged by her parents and is expected to be self-sacrificing, accommodating to the needs of the family, and the keeper and bearer of Indian tradition (Kundu et al., 2005). She is prepared for this life through being raised since childhood to be tolerant, adaptive, religious, affectionate, and to most highly value the family (Kundu et al., 2005). It would be unheard of for an East Indian couple to not want to have children (Dattilio et al., 2005).

Arranged marriages are tied to religious beliefs and are the norm in India and for East Indians in America (Baptiste, 2005). It would be seen as a rejection of family and culture for an East Indian woman, even from the affluent and educated classes, to refuse an arranged marriage, to date socially, or marry for love (Medora et al., 2003). Dating or marrying non-East Indians, and even outside ones' regional or religious background, is generally considered completely unacceptable (Poulsen, 2009). Serious, long-term romantic relationships outside of marriage are rare in Indian society and are socially frowned upon (Natarajan et al., 2005). This is of concern because research supports that East Indian young adults whose parents had a love marriage rated their *families as stronger* than young adults whose parents had an arranged marriage (Medora et al., 2003).

This discussion shows that East Indian men enjoy greater social entitlements and privileges than women, who are devalued in everyday life (Baptiste, 2005; Dattilio et al., 2005). This makes it difficult for East Indian women to develop a positive identity, which is important because positive identity is associated with a generally positive sense of well-being, psychological adjustment, self-esteem, and more successful integration of Indian and American culture, particularly for East Indian teenage girls (Kundu et al., 2005). Traditional East Indian cultural values make it difficult for East Indian women to adjust to an American society that encourages women to be independent and autonomous (Poulsen, 2009).

Discussion Question: *Traditional East Indian societies have been shown to subordinate women. How would this present challenges for a family therapist working with an East Indian family?*

Now that I have discussed the father and mother's role in traditional East Indian society, I will discuss parenting practices. East Indian children are expected to obey their parents and behave in ways that reflect well upon the family (Medora et al., 2003; Baptiste, 2005). Problem behaviors include changes in dietary habits, marrying across racial and class lines, drinking alcohol, females wearing revealing clothing, teenage pregnancy, using contraception, children not having pre-arranged marriages, and pre-marital co-habitation (Baptiste, 2005). Within the East Indian community, parents are held responsible for their children's behavior and are criticized for their failings as parents by the larger East Indian community (Baptiste, 2005). East Indian children in therapy often complain of the social restrictions on their behavior and how this places them in a bind between doing what they must do to succeed in America and their parents' desires for them to remain, in all ways, Indian (Baptiste, 2005).

In India, adolescents who are born in America and raised by 1st generation East Indian parents are referred to as *ABCD*: American-Born, Confused *Desis*, a term that refers to people from India (Poulsen, 2009). The implication of this terminology is that American-born East Indian children will be difficult to parent and will be confused about their identities, misunderstand their culture, and create problems for themselves and their families (Poulsen, 2009). This label minimizes how genuinely difficult it is for East Indian adolescents to simultaneously manage their parents' demands and the demands of their adolescent socio-culture, and overlooks the fact that successfully traversing two cultural worlds is often an enriching experience (Poulsen, 2009; Dattilio et al., 2005).

Kundu et al. (2005) report that: "Children of immigrant parents have one foot planted in their parents' traditional home life and the other foot planted in the world outside the front door. The journey to adulthood and finding one's place in the world is difficult enough, but children of immigrants must also find an ethnic identity that will harmonize one culture with the other" (p. 247). Minority adolescents usually develop their ethnic identities during late adolescence (Kundu et al., 2005).

In East Indian families, adolescence may not be recognized as distinct phase of separation and individuation as it is in America (Kundu et al., 2005). Rather, East Indian households may expect developing adolescents to clarify their expectations within the household and to take on more responsibilities (Kundu et al., 2005). Conformity is equated with loyalty, while separation-individuation is seen as a rejection of parents and culture (Baptiste, 2005). Parents may attempt to preserve their native culture and its influence on their family by repressing children's individuation through strict and rigid rules, particularly for adolescent daughters in regards to dating and the opposite sex (Baptiste, 2005; Poulsen, 2009). East Indian parents in America may be even more traditional in their parenting practices than their counterparts in India (Poulsen, 2009).

East Indian parents generally do not see children as capable of making sound judgments (Medora et al., 2003). There is more of a rigid hierarchy which does not encourage or promote adolescent independence (Medora et al., 2003). This often leads children to rebel, verbally retaliate, or behave passive-aggressively (Medora et al., 2003).

Indian families generally do not emphasize open expressions of love and affection and, instead, emphasize age and experience (Medora et al., 2003). Most Indian parents prefer a certain distance so that children respect their age, wisdom, power, and authority (Medora et al., 2003). This may be particularly difficult for Indians of traditional college age who may desire autonomy and freedom, though also emotional support, friendly advice, or a hug (Medora et al., 2003). Indian adolescents typically do not share their feelings with their parents because they feel their parents won't listen, understand, or help (Medora et al., 2003). When asked by researchers, *what would you want to see changed in your family*, Indian children most often reported wanting their parents to be more open-minded and consultative, and also desiring greater freedom and independence (Medora et al., 2003). The family and parenting structure and desire for more rights amongst East Indian children is generally consistent with the desires of children in other Asian immigrant populations (Kwak et al., 2001).

East Indian parents expect to have a high degree of control over their children's social environment, including monitoring their friends, particularly non-East Indian friends (Poulsen, 2009). Adolescents in America tend to be socialized by their peers, which Indian parents may see as corruptive influences and respond by more closely monitoring the youth until marriage (Kundu et al., 2005).

Indian parents also tend to have a strong desire for their children to become highly educated and economically successful (Baptiste, 2005). This often leads East Indian children to strive to succeed in order to please their parents, often at the expense of other developmental needs, which intensifies the normative stress of adolescence and young adulthood (Baptiste, 2005). This may lead East Indian children to experience mental health issues, which often results in families being referred for family therapy (Baptiste, 2005). East Indian children in therapy often complain that their parents only value their educational and financial success and disregard their personal happiness and growth (Baptiste, 2005).

Discussion Question: *It is important for family therapists to be aware of who they tend to ally with so as not to develop imbalanced therapeutic relationships with participating family members. As you read about traditional East Indian parenting values, would you be more likely to ally with? East Indian parents or children? How might your natural alliance be helpful* <u>*and/or*</u> *harmful to the therapeutic work?*

____

____

____

____

____

____

____

MULTI-DIMENSIONAL FAMILY THERAPY

MDFT is a traditional family therapeutic approach that has been tested in federally-funded research projects since 1985, was developed from clinical research, and was refined through therapy studies (Liddle et al., 2005; Liddle, 1995). It is an evidence-based, modular, and comprehensive approach to improving adolescents' psychosocial functioning through interventions in *the four domains:* (e.g. dimensions): the adolescent, parent, family interaction, and extra-familial (Liddle et al., 2006; Liddle, 1995).

The adolescent domain encapsulates the adolescents' academic and social functioning, including adolescents' abilities to communicate effectively, grades, behavior at school, and problem solving skills (Liddle et al., 2005). The parent domain denotes parenting skills and practices, including age-appropriate rules for the adolescent and the parents' disciplinary enforcement of those rules (Liddle et al., 2005). The family interactional domain pertains to interfamilial communication and the strength of familial relationships (Liddle et al., 2005). The extra-familial domain refers to the relative health of family members' interactions with outside systems such as schools, recreational agencies, and juvenile justice providers (Hogue et al., 2006). The sum total of which is theorized to predict the relative health of adolescent development (Diamond et al., 1999). This shows that MDFT also has roots in ecological theory and developmental psychology (Shelef et al., 2005; Hogue et al., 2006).

Adolescent substance abuse is conceptualized as a deviation from healthy, adaptive development and indicative of impaired family functioning (Liddle et al., 2005). Improving functioning in the four domains through family-focused interventions is therefore expected to strengthen the family, which will decrease substance abuse and place adolescents on healthier developmental trajectories (Shelef et al., 2005). MDFT has been found to be effective with adolescent substance abusers who were: younger and older, white, African-American, and Latino, referred from the criminal justice system, lower income, and had more severe co-occurring disorders (Liddle et al., 2009; Henderson et al., 2010).

Discussion Question: *Would you expect MDFT to be an acceptable model of practice for traditional East Indian families? Why or why not?*

THE FAMILY THERAPY CASE OF SANJITA

I will now present Sanjita's case in stages and will summarize the most clinically significant interchanges and themes. This framework will help to create a coherent narrative of what will be shown to be a complicated family history, presentation, and treatment episode. I will present the details of the family history as the details were made known to me and to transcribe what really happened in the therapy, which will give my reader a sense of *what it was like to be with the family at different points in the case*, a subjective-emotional factor that I have found to be very informative to family therapeutic work with culturally diverse populations with significant risk factors. All treatment data that can be disguised (without compromising the integrity of the case) will be disguised so as to protect Sanjita and her families' confidentiality.

Stage One: Alliance-Building

I was a family therapist in private practice in metropolitan Miami, FL and worked mostly with lower-income families on a sliding-scale fee basis. I received a call from a local emergency room reporting that 14-year-old Sanjita had attempted homicide and suicide while under the influence of alcohol. The referent triage nurse reported that Sanjita had just completed medical treated for alcohol poisoning as her blood alcohol level was 0.23, nearly three times the legal limit to drive. She was reported to have climbed out of her bedroom window without her parents' permission in the middle of the night two nights prior. Around three o'clock in the morning, she burst back through the front door of the family home, crying and screaming incoherently. Her mother awoke first and responded by slapping Sanjita across the face, which lead Sanjita to reach for a nearby kitchen knife. While being quickly subdued by her mother and father, Sanjita's 19 year old sister called the police. Before the police could arrive, Sanjita tried to stab both her mother and herself. Though none of these details that Sanjita told to the emergency medical staff were reported to the police, which coincides with previously discussed East Indian cultural values for privacy and behaving in ways that do not bring shame to the family (Baptiste, 2005). Sanjita was admitted to the emergency room for alcohol detoxification and no police report was filed. While in the hospital, Sanjita told medical staff that her families' *real problem* was her father and mother's chronic marriage conflict and daily abuse of marijuana.

Having received a contact phone number from the referent nurse, I telephoned the family and introduced myself to the father as a family therapist in private practice. I informed him that I had received information from the emergency room staff that his daughter Sanjita had been in the hospital with alcohol poisoning. I summarized my understanding of the incident as "quite a rough night," offering my condolences and inquiring as to whether the father may be interested in family therapy. I explained that family therapeutic services had been helpful in similar cases in the past and that family therapy was usually preferable to individual therapy with adolescent substance abusers because involved adults needed to "be on the same page." The father readily agreed. I prescribed these interventions so as to pre-emptively address what might be the father's ideas about referring Sanjita to individual behavior-changing therapy and to build professional credibility, both of which are discussed by Baptiste (2005) as potential concerns of East Indian families.

The father sounded understandably anxious, which lead me not to ask a lot of informational questions either over the phone or in person. My experience has often been that standard question-answer intake formats are often experienced by clients-of-color as intrusive. I concluded that Sanjita and her family would tell me the details I really needed to know when I really needed to know them. It was particularly important for me to begin allying with Sanjita's father because alliance with the parents tends to predict therapeutic engagement in family therapy (Shelef et al., 2005).

Three days after the initial phone conversation, the father brought Sanjita to treatment. He was a heavier set man who looked approximately 60 years old, with a beard and turban, leaning on a cane, lighter brown skin, and deep, hollow set eyes that seemed to see only what was necessary. Sanjita was thin-framed and had shorter dark brown hair and a contemptuous look on her face, smiling at me politely in greeting, though quickly returning to a sullen demeanor, seeming quite uncertain and unsettled about whatever was in store for her. The father informed me that his wife and 19 year old daughter Shazia were working, and his 11 year old daughter Nalini was at home studying.

As we sat down, the father began to inform me at length of Sanjita's failings, including her poor grades, history of arguing with her teachers, and incorrigible behavior at home. It sounded almost as if he wanted to therapy to "fix" Sanjita's behavior, which is consistent with Baptiste's (2005) report that East Indian parents often bring their adolescents to therapy with the hope that therapy will return the adolescent to Indian culture-normative behavior.

Discussion Question: *At this point in the therapy, who are you finding yourself allying with in Sanjita's family and how might that be helpful and/or harmful to the therapeutic work?*

I found myself growing irritated at the father, though tried to calm myself as I glanced over at Sanjita and noticed that she also looked irritated, which informed me that I was beginning to ally more with her. This is of concern because allying more strongly with adolescents than the parents in family therapy has been found to predict early termination of adolescent substance abuse treatment and has also been found to exacerbate East Indian parent-child conflicts (Shelef et al., 2005; Baptiste, 2005).

At the earliest possible juncture, I commented that Sanjita "looked like she wanted to say something," so as to give her a voice but in a way that might did not seem like I was encouraging her to argue with her father. My technique coincides with Dattilio et al.'s (2005) finding that it is important for East Indians' family therapists to not encourage adolescent independence too early in the treatment, but rather to seek solutions that are culturally appropriate. The authors elaborate that family therapy with any family whose culture varies from the therapists' culture requires not only cultural awareness, but also a collaborative approach that allows the families' cultural beliefs to inform the treatment goals and process.

As can be expected, Sanjita attempted to refute everything her father said, contending that her grades and behavior had improved recently and that her family members' constant arguing was "the real problem." I inquired about whether the verbal sparring I had just witnessed between Sanjita and her father was consistent with the dynamics they frequently experienced at home, wanting to add that no wonder Sanjita ended up in the hospital, though resisting the impulse to potentially take sides. My intervention was consistent with research-based recommendations that family therapists help adolescent substance abusers and their families *enact* their longstanding disagreements, though the therapeutic focus should be shifted from the content of the arguments to family members' deeper feelings about the familial relationship itself (Liddle et al., 2005; Diamond et al., 1996).

Sanjita and her father readily agreed that the constant quarrels were a problem and that something needed to change, though quickly lapsed back into disagreements about school work and house hold chores. This interchange occurred repeatedly over the course of my first few sessions with the family. Sanjita and her father seemed most interested in the content of their disagreements and I obliged by attempting to teach effective communication skills and re-framing less functional interchanges in ways that illuminated the family members' underlying good intentions, cognitive interventions that are consistent with the CBT approaches to family therapy discussed by Datillio et al. (2005) and East Indian family strengths (Medora et al., 2003). This deferment to the families' implicitly preferred treatment approach speaks to Baptiste's (2005) recommendation that therapists accept East Indians' family problems as they are defined by the family.

I also noted to myself that substance abuse was not brought up by Sanjita's father in spite of Sanjita having been hospitalized for an alcohol overdose. My experience has been that this sense of secrecy about substance abuse suggests that the problem may be severe, which I definitely sensed in this case, though I hypothesized that bringing substance abuse up early in the treatment would be intrusive and therefore better left to the family members to bring up on their own.

Stage Two: The Truth Coming Out

At my request, Sanjita's father began to bring his entire family to family therapy sessions, including his wife and three daughters. His wife and eldest daughter were both darker skinned, slender, and attractive, with long, jet-black hair and inquisitive eyes, and were wearing extravagant good jewelry. The youngest daughter was heavier set, wearing brighter clothes, and was sullen and prone to looking disparagingly when her parents talked. I informed the family of five that I been meeting with Sanjita and her father, together, though was eager to hear everyone's "take on what was going on in the family," which is consistent with Baptiste's (2005) finding that American therapists instinctively move quickly to create egalitarianism in patriarchal East Indian families.

The father answered my invitation by informing me of his concerns about each family member, one by one, including his wife/their daughter's mother. I noted to myself that criticizing his wife in front of their children sent the children a structurally inappropriate message about their mother's place in the family, which I know now to be consistent with East Indian cultural values.

10 or so minutes into his disclosure, without interruption, my irritation was becoming intolerable. Just then, Sanjita and Shazia collectively interrupted him to complain about his constant criticisms of them. The father defended his reports on the basis that his elder daughters were doing poorly in school and regularly failed to do their assigned household

chores. Looking back on it, the girls arguing with their father (particularly in front of a non-East Indian stranger) was outside the boundaries of traditional East Indian family values, a breakdown of family structure which is consistent with the effects of chronic substance abuse (Ruiz et al., 2007).

As the girls began to argue with their father, the mother joined the conversation in support of her husband, adding that the girls tended to ignore their house hold responsibilities and leave them to her to complete after a long days' work as an attorney. This communication is an example of Baptiste's (2005) report that East Indian parents often use guilt and shame to keep their children focused on family obligations.

Sanjita and Shazia responded to their mother by complaining that she was only interested in maintaining the house hold and making money, and did not speak to them unless she had orders to give, which the youngest daughter Nalinee agreed with by nodding. The girls' mutual concern is consistent with the concerns of East Indian youth who were surveyed about their family problems and reported that their parents are more interested in their (various forms of) performance than their happiness (Medora et al., 2003). By this point, I was hypothesizing that family conflict was a primary risk factor for Sanjita's alcohol abuse and was therefore *the treatment priority*, which is consistent with research on traditional family therapeutic approaches to adolescent substance abuse treatment (Liddle et al., 2005).

Sanjita defended herself against her mother's criticisms by interjecting that the *real problem* was that her mother and father were always fighting if they were not smoking marijuana together. In newfound interest, I sat back further in my chair and observed more closely. The parents looked noticeably uncomfortable as Sanjita more intensely scolded them, particularly her mother, for giving her directions to be sober and act responsible in ways that the parents themselves did not follow.

Discussion Question: *In what ways does Sanjita's families' presentation coincide with traditional East Indian cultural values and in what ways are the family members' behaviors out of cultural baseline? What are some of your ideas about things you might say to them in family sessions so as to increase family functioning?*

Although in silent agreement with Sanjita's position, I felt it necessary to interrupt the chastising of her parents so that the parents would not potentially associate their experience in therapy with being disrespected by their children in front of an outsider, a concern that is fundamentally consistent with East Indian cultural values and the principles of traditional family therapy (Baptiste, 2005; J. Kirk, personal communication, 06/10/11).[1] I followed my intuition to inform the family of my professional opinion (based on similar cases in the past) that Sanjita's recovery depended on them *becoming a sober family*. This is a family-focused treatment intervention that I have sometimes found to be effective in similar cases. This appeal to the family system as a unit that was capable of changing is consistent with research findings in support of orienting treatment to East Indian family strengths (Poulsen, 2009; Medora et al., 2003).

All family members seemed noticeably uncomfortable and, for the first time, no one looked particularly eager to speak in session. Each family member took turns downplaying his or her own individual use and to stress that other family members' behavior was the real problem, not the substance abuse.

I responded by educating the family about how family conflicts are often a symptom of substance abuse and, based on an intuition, asked the father directly if he was open to being sober to set an example for the rest of the family. Looking anxious though also receptive, the father agreed. He may have accepted my intervention because it reinforced his position as the head of household and decision-maker, which is consistent with traditional East Indian cultural values and traditional family therapeutic principles (Medora et al., 2003; J. Kirk, personal communication, 8/20/11). The psycho-educational component of my interventions is also mentioned in research studies as being potentially helpful to East Indian families (Poulsen, 2009). It is possible that the father agreed to be sober out of deference to me (which would coincide with traditional Hindu values for being agreeable and avoiding conflict) and it was also difficult to tell whether he would remain sober as promised. Nevertheless, his agreement to be sober in front of his family, in and of itself, sent Sanjita an important message about sobriety.

Over the next couple months, I tended to begin family sessions by inquiring about Sanjita and her father's sobriety, encouraged them to talk openly about what sobriety felt like, and encouraged family members to comment on what it was like to see Sanjita and the father sober. This focus on sobriety as paramount is consistent with research that supports that interventions with East Indian families should be directive, clear, and focused on a limited number of behavior changes (Baptiste, 2005; Poulsen, 2009).

Family members continued to quarrel openly in session, though became progressively more receptive to my attempts to teach effective communication skills. The family members' in-session quarrels decreased in intensity over time, which may suggest that they were also quarreling less in the home. Interestingly, research findings support of relationship between decreased family conflict and decreased *adolescent* substance abuse (Shelef et al., 2005), though my paper also shows that decreased *parental substance abuse* has a relationship with decreased family conflict.

So as to provide additional recovery-support for sobering family members, I regularly checked-in with the father over the phone, and tried to connect Sanjita, her elder sister, and her mother to individual therapy with female therapists. The father responded positively to my efforts, though the three women terminated individual therapy after only two or three sessions. Research supports that East Indians tend not to take female therapists seriously and

[1] Kirk is an LCSW and structural family therapist with over 30 years of experience treating families of adolescent substance abusers.

may not engage, particularly if the female therapist attempts to connect with them in a feminist-empowering way that clashes with East Indian cultural values (Baptiste, 2005).

Discussion Question: *What are some of your ideas about how you might attempt to be helpful to Sanjita and the women in her family, at this stage in the treatment, without challenging their cultural values?*

____

____

____

____

____

____

____

Stage Three: Growth and Maintenance

As we started the fourth month of treatment, the father requested to see me individually. I agreed to see him because, although he was not the identified client, individual-conjoint work with the parents is an essential part of adolescent substance abuse treatment (Liddle et al., 2005). The father informed me that he had "mostly" abstained from abusing marijuana, though his wife had been retaliating by refusing to have sex with him. The father did not seem angry, but more hopeless, possibly in regards to the totality of his families' issues. My sense was that this reaction was evidence that he had in fact decreased his substance abuse. Contrastingly, I would have associated a blaming-angry response to his wife with non-decreased substance abuse. These hypotheses' are based on my experiences with men-of-color who are in romantic relationships in early recovery where ongoing substance abusers more frequently tend to engage in blaming behavior and avoid underlying depressive feelings. Sanjita's father may have also felt hopeless about the deeper issue of losing his absolute authority and dominance in the home, which Poulsen (2009) noted to be a common struggle for East Indian fathers in America.

I validated the father for being vulnerable with me, and encouraged him to tell me more about what had been transpiring with his wife in the home since he had been "mostly sober." He presented a very detailed, long and complicated narrative of the families' conflicts, which included an acknowledgement that he often swore at his wife and had been yelling at her in front of their children ever since the beginning of their arranged marriage 10 years prior. He reported that he and his wife concurred that they were not happy together, though were committed to staying together for the children. At the conclusion of the session, I asked him to bring his entire family to the next session.

In the next family session, the girls regularly interrupted their mother when she was speaking and spoke to her in a mocking, disrespectful tone. I asked the entire family where the girls learned that it was appropriate to disrespect their mother. No one responded, though everyone present (of course) knew that the girls learned to disrespect their mother from observing their father. This interchange supports Baptiste's (2005) report that American therapists sometimes attempt to encourage a wife and children to collectively challenge the father's authority, which the wife and children are likely to resist. Their passive resistance is consist with Medora et al.'s (2003) report that East Indian family members tend to suppress emotions and express them subtly and indirectly.

In subsequent individual-conjoint meetings with the father, I asked him if he was open to supporting his wife by intervening when their daughters were disrespectful. In response, he changed the subject and frequently did so when I attempted traditional family therapeutic interventions that I now know to conflict with traditional East Indian cultural values. The repeated failures of such interventions support Baptiste's (2005) report that East Indians' beliefs about gender are inexorably tied to religion and any therapeutic effort to change these beliefs will therefore be resisted.

Discussion Question: *How would you reconcile your ethical responsibility to empower disenfranchised populations (e.g. women) and your ethical responsibility to practice in a way that is respectful and honoring of cultural values that you may not agree with (including traditional East Indian values for women being of a subordinate status)?*

Stage Four: The Father Taking Charge

In the first five months of therapy, I informed the father of who I wanted to be present for family sessions so that I could structure the sessions in a way that would support various interventions that required only certain family members to be present. For example, I would only discuss issues of discipline or parenting with the father in individual sessions or with both parents (when the mother was not working) because it would not be appropriate to attempt to negotiate parenting strategies in front of the children (J. Kirk, personal communication, 04/10/10).

After five months of therapy, I advised the father to make his own decisions about who would attend each session. This intervention was designed to reinforce that he was a competent father and house hold authority, which he demonstrated to a greater extent after committing to decrease his substance abuse. As an example of his progress, the father interrupted his family members less frequently in therapy sessions and, often, attempted to more softly negotiate with them rather than telling them what to do. Now that I think about it, these improvements in therapy may have been suggestive of improvements made in the home, though probably to a lesser extent as my relatively longer standing therapeutic presence may have had a grounding effect on the father's affect while he was in therapy.

The father obliged my request for him to structure family sessions as he saw fit, and returned to bringing only Sanjita to sessions. Looking back on it, this was an appropriate decision as Sanjita was the family member with the most significant risk factors (e.g. hospitalizations). Furthermore, it is possible that I became distracted from the main treatment priorities by the family members ongoing conflicts, which the father may have even anticipated and therefore only brought Sanjita to sessions in the beginning.

In more recent sessions with Sanjita, the father tended to express lengthy concern about her not doing chores and speaking loudly and disrespectfully when she was asked to. Sanjita would usually respond in session by groaning loudly and rolling her eyes. The father's complaints tended to be long and tangential, which Sanjita could only listen to in session for so long before reacting. I often intervened by summarizing the father's parental directives and re-framing his lengthier statements in terms of their ultimately good parenting objectives. This is consistent with the parenting skill building principle of MDFT and research in support of interventions that help East Indian parents communicate their expectations clearly to the adolescent (Poulsen, 2009; Liddle et al, 2005). Often, these interventions were only minimally effective, possibly because the father's capacity to process and make use of new information was diminished by longstanding marijuana abuse, which is consistent with my experience with long term marijuana abusers.

After another month of the aforementioned parent-child sessions, the father called me and requested that Sanjita be randomly drug tested. I obliged this request as we had discussed testing as a possible adjunct treatment earlier in treatment. Research also supports random urinalysis for adolescent substance abusers (Liddle et al., 2005).

I inquired about whether the father would be comfortable with me informing Sanjita that she had been selected to test when she arrived at the next family therapy session and then accompanying her to the testing laboratory across the street. I explained that this would provide Sanjita with an opportunity to disclose any past drug abuse to me so that I could coach her on bringing the drug abuse up with her father directly. I added that adolescents, in my experience, were usually reluctant to inform their parents about drug abuse, which is why the coaching would be necessary. I elaborated that, if Sanjita disclosed a positive screen, she should not be required to test provided she was willing to disclose her drug abuse history to her father. I also explained that, if she disclosed drug abuse honestly to her father, it would be helpful to her recovery for her father to acknowledge her for being honest even when being honest would get her into trouble. I prefaced this by saying that acknowledging her honesty did not mean she would go on without consequences, though I also recommended that the father non-punitively respond to her admission of drug abuse by increasing house hold structure and parental monitoring. I added that, if Sanjita tested clean, she needed to be positively reinforced. My recommendations in this interchange are consistent with research findings in support of teaching effective communication and problem solving skills to adolescent substance abusers *and* East Indian families, and building professional credibility through demonstrating treatment knowledge (Baptiste, 2005; Poulsen, 2009; Liddle et al., 2005). The father acknowledged my points and agreed to this plan, which offers some support for my position that East Indian families may be receptive to the multi-dimensional family therapeutic approach to adolescent substance abuse treatment, largely, because the interventions attempt to reinforce parental authority and help adolescents learn social and problem solving skills that are acceptable in East Indian culture.

When Sanjita and her father arrived at their next family session, I informed Sanjita that she would be taking a drug test. Sanjita uneasily agreed and we began to walk to the testing laboratory across the street. She began to ask questions about testing procedures and toxicology detection. I informed her that it was difficult to predict test results in a general way as testing results varied depending on ones' body composition and other personal factors, adding that her father was likely to respond far better if she honestly and candidly admitted drug abuse rather than denying drug abuse and potentially being contradicted by the test results. She then asked what I would advise her to tell her father. I suggested she tell him *everything*, which she agreed to do as we returned to my office. Her agreement provides support for recommendation that individual work with adolescents focus on teaching them problem solving communication strategies so as to provide them with alternatives to acting out behaviors.

Sanjita fearfully informed her father of having experimented with cocaine approximately a year ago, and drinking alcohol and smoking marijuana "regularly." So as to remind Sanjita's father of our plan in a way that was structurally appropriate given his daughter being in the room, I validated Sanjita for being honest about her drug abuse even when being honest was likely to get her into trouble.

Sanjita's father shook his head in silence and looked down at his feet remorsefully. Sanjita looked out the window and back to her father in a way that suggested (what I would call) healthy guilt.

The father broke a long silence by openly suspected that Sanjita's mother may have been influencing Sanjita's drug abuse and began to criticize her (the mother). Sanjita angrily responded that marijuana and alcohol intensified the pleasurable feelings she incurred from having sex with her boyfriend, a provocative way of defending her mother that both her father and I were too shocked to respond to. This disclosure was particularly shocking in light of the conservative East Indian cultural views about dating and pre-marital sex, particularly for teenage girls (Natarajan et al., 2005).

In spite of this last interchange, we ended the session with my feeling hopeful in light of Sanjita being honest with her father about her substance abuse and sexual relations. My experience with adolescent substance abusers has been that there is a relationship between adolescent honesty to parents and decreased substance abuse. Unfortunately, the families' insurance denied services due to eligibility reasons just at this point when I felt that we were finally getting somewhere.

Discussion Question: *If you were Sanjita's families' therapist and were able to continue meeting with them, what would be your most immediate treatment priorities?*

____

____

____

____

CONCLUSION AND IMPLICATIONS FOR THE FUTURE

The forced termination of treatment was disappointing, though I acknowledged to myself that the family had made some significant gains. Most notably, family members' experienced intermittent periods of improved communication and decreased family conflict and the father decreased his substance abuse. I was worried about whether the family was capable of independently maintaining their gains, though resolved myself to the spiritual challenge of believing they were ready to go on without me. The father and I reviewed key areas of family progress, developed a transition plan that included emergency service contacts, and said our heart-felt goodbyes'.

I worked with this family before undertaking research on East Indians and now find myself wishing that I knew then what I know now about East Indian culture and recommendations for treatment. My intuitions and training in traditional family therapy sometimes lead me to intervene in ways that coincidentally aligned with East Indian cultural values and the core principles of MDFT. The research I more recently did on East Indians lead to helpful insights about why my interventions worked or did not work, as well as ideas about new and potentially helpful interventions. In particular, it might have been helpful for me to ask the family members to talk about their experiences in India, what immigration was like for them, and how they might reconcile the differences between their native East Indian values and host-American values, as is noted by Poulsen (2009) to be a best practice. These psychodynamic interventions might have more deeply addressed the family conflicts that I addressed on a more surface level through improving *communication skills* and decreasing *substance abuse*, which could be conceptualized as symptoms of underlying cultural conflicts.

It is highly possible that therapy with Sanjita's family (as with other East Indian families) could never completely change their beliefs about gender and parenting, though my sense is that my work with Sanjita's father helped him modulate his role as the undisputed, authoritarian head of household. This last finding, as well as the conceptual relationship I demonstrated between East Indians' cultural clash and family conflict, and between family conflict and substance abuse, makes me wonder if substance abuse might be a more significant problem for East Indian families (parents and children) than what might be assumed by peer-reviewed literature making little to no mention of it. It is possible that substance abuse has not been discussed as a significant risk factor for East Indians because East Indians underreport for fear of bringing dishonor to their families and larger East Indian community. Further study is needed to ascertain the extent of substance abuse problems in East Indian communities and the reliability of family therapeutic treatment approaches.

Chapter 7

STRENGTHENING VULNERABLE FAMILIES THROUGH MULTIDIMENSIONAL FAMILY THERAPY*

INTRODUCTION

Adolescent substance abuse is a social problem that is deserving of greater priority in the national public health agenda (Liddle et al., 2009). It associates with adolescent antisocial behavior, poor academic performance, low self-esteem, mental health symptomology, and problems in adulthood with adjustment, employment, and interpersonal relationships (Liddle, Rowe et al., 2009; Shelef et al., 2005; Kilpatrick et al., 2000). Substance abuse among adolescents is particularly risky because of the relative brevity between onset of first use and the *addiction*, at which point psychopathology that associates with substance abuse becomes more intense, ingrained, and difficult to treat (Ruiz et al., 2007). This underscores the importance of developing preventative interventions (Liddle et al., 2009).

Discussion Question: *Given what you have just read about adolescent substance abuse, re-consider the previous discussion question about your therapeutic objectives for Sanjita's family. Would you change your answer? If so, please describe.*

____

____

____

____

____

Evidence-based literature supports that many treatments can help adolescents t decrease their substance abuse and related behavior problems, including group therapy, ecological family therapy, cognitive-behavioral therapy (CBT), and *multidimensional family therapy*

* A version of this chapter has been accepted for publication by *Child & Youth Work*, a journal that is part of the Taylor & Francis Group. It has been expanded in an effort to encourage wider dissemination of research on the subject.

(MDFT) (Liddle et al., 2009; Henderson et al., 2010; Chasin et al., 2006; Becker et al., 2006). The latter model will be the subject of this chapter because I have found that intuitively integrating its core principles in family therapeutic approaches to treating adolescent substance abusers has often resulted in positive therapeutic outcomes, particularly for highly vulnerable and disenfranchised families. Later, I will demonstrate this through a case presentation.

MDFT in Theory

The multi-dimensional family therapy approach targets four interdependent *domains*: the adolescent, parent, family interaction, and extra-familial (Liddle et al., 2009). The adolescent domain involves psycho educating the adolescent about social skills and relapse prevention skills. The parent domain involves the teaching of parenting skills, including limit setting and discipline, though also increasing emotional responsiveness. The latter, family interaction domain focuses on strengthening family members' relationships and increasing interpersonal problem solving skills. The extra-familial domain pertains to collateral therapeutic work with outside service providers, including juvenile justice and school officials. Research speculates that interventions in the latter three domains are responsible for significant amounts of positive change in the adolescent because the interventions ultimately change the parents, and therefore change the adolescent by proxy (Henderson et al., 2010).

The MDFT therapist may meet with one parent or both parents, the adolescent individually, or the entire family (Shelef et al., 2005). Different session structures may support alliance building with different members (Shelef et al., 2005). Therapeutic alliance with the parents most strongly predicts engagement in the early stages of treatment, while alliance with the adolescent is the strongest predictor of therapeutic outcome (Shelef et al., 2005; Flicker et al., 2008).

Research consistently supports that MDFT leads to considerable decreases in adolescent substance abuse and related behavior problems, even in co-occurring adolescents who tend (Liddle et al., 2009). This finding has held true in cases of youth with more severe co-occurring psychiatric symptomology, who are frequently the most difficult to engage and treat (Henderson et al., 2010).

Discussion Question: *Given what you have just read about the finer points of multi-dimensional family therapy, do any new interventions come to mind that you might have liked to try in sessions with Sanjita's family? If so, please describe them.*

____

____

____

____

MDFT in Practice: The Case of Johnny

Now that I have presented background information on adolescent substance abuse and MDFT as an evidence-based therapeutic approach to treatment, I will present the family therapy case of *Johnny*. All case material that is not germane to important outcomes has been disguised so as to protect confidentiality. I will show that intuitively practicing in alignment with the principles of MDFT helped Johnny decrease his substance abuse, improve his academic performance, and inspire positive parenting changes in his foster parents. Admittedly, I didn't know exactly what model I was following until long after termination. In session, I generally followed my intuitions about how to intervene. It was often helpful to meet with the family members individually and build relationships with them through empathic listening. Once I felt that I had built meaningful alliances, interventions targeting communication and problem solving skills were more effective. As predicted in MDFT theory, related improvements contributed to Johnny's aforementioned gains.

As I described in previous chapters of this book, positive outcomes inspired me to search for a clinical theory that could explain what happened in Johnny's family therapy. Through my research, I concluded that my approach to Johnny's treatment most strongly coincided with MDFT.

The Family History

Johnny's immediate family consisted of his foster father, Mr. Jones, his foster mother, Mrs. Jones, and his biological half-sister Katrina. They were a lower-income Irish American family who resided in a public housing community in West Virginia. Mr. Jones was a retired electrician with chronic back pain. Mrs. Jones was a lifelong homemaker. It is important for the larger subject matter (of treating vulnerable populations) to present the case of a lower-income, rural Caucasian family based on my experience that they have fairly unique and generally less understood limitations.

Johnny and his sister were both foster children soon after birth because their biological parents were chronic alcoholics who failed to provide adequate supervision. Mr. and Mrs. Jones described Johnny and Katrina as remaining together throughout a series of temporary foster placements. In each placement, they were returned to the system due to chronic lying and defiant behavior.

Mr. and Mrs. Jones had previously cared for four other foster children over the last 10 years, though reported experiencing Johnny and Katrina as particularly exhausting of their collective patience. Katrina was consistently on the honor roll for academic excellence, though was nevertheless quarrelsome at home. Johnny consistently received D's and F's on his report cards and was suspected to be abusing drugs and/or alcohol.

Mr. Jones requested treatment for Johnny after a recent suicide attempt. Johnny had overdosed on over-the-counter pills and was hospitalized for one week. Before I could ask any questions about Johnny's suicide attempt, Mr. Jones changed the subject to Johnny's behavior problems and poor grades. So as to support the building of an alliance with Mr. Jones, I elected not to ask a lot of informational questions. Instead, I learned the family history over the organic course of the case.

Discussion Question: *At this point in the case, who do you find yourself allying with in Johnny's family and how might your natural alliance be helpful* <u>*and/or*</u> *harmful to the therapeutic work?*

____

____

____

____

____

THE FIRST SESSION

The family presented to my office for their first session three days later. Mr. Jones leaned heavily on his right side as they entered my office, holding his back in demonstration of ongoing pain. He was unkempt and averted eye contact. He walked slowly, with each family member seeming to make a considerable effort to keep pace with him and to remain standing until he was seated. Johnny made a noticeable effort to sit as far away from Mr. Jones as he could. He was skinny, dressed all in black, and wore sullen, angry-teenager look on his face.

As I expected, Mr. Jones immediately began to tell me about Johnny's poor grades and defiant behavior, as if Johnny wasn't in the room. I was more concerned about Johnny's recent suicide attempt, though I decided to let Mr. Jones ventilate his concerns and listen for a pattern family dynamic.

Meanwhile, Mrs. Jones seemed to shrink back into her chair, looking embarrassed and sorrowful. She wore plain, older clothing, and also looked very tired. She sat between Mr. Jones on her left and their foster children on her right. Katrina sat particularly close to her, with Johnny on Katrina's right. It seemed like Katrina and Mrs. Jones were very connected in their own way and that Johnny was subtly trying to disappear from Mr. Jones' purview. I sensed that this physical arrangement might be a clue to underlying family dynamics.

Five minutes into Mr. Jones' tirade, I could feel Johnny's annoyance. I gently interrupted so as to ask Johnny to share his experience of what was happening at home and at school. This inclusion of the teenager's perspective is consistent with Flicker, Turner, Waldron, and Brody et al.'s (2008) recommendation that family therapists intervene when parents engage in excessive blaming of the adolescent early in the therapy. Enthusiastically, Johnny discredited everything that Mr. Jones had said about him. In response, Mr. Jones interrupted Johnny and re-asserted his position with enough of a forceful undertone to quiet Johnny's objections. Mrs. Jones breathed heavily, looking down at the floor as if she badly needed a vacation.

Katrina suddenly bolted upright in her chair, taking a closer look at Mr. Jones out of the corner of her eye. Before I could interrupt Mr. Jones, Katrina began to curse him belligerently in defense of her brother. Mrs. Jones seemed to shrink even further back into the chair. Johnny scowled as if to say, "here we go again."

In order to prevent family feuding, I interrupted Katrina and re-framed Mr. Jones' concerns about Johnny in ways that emphasized his ultimately good parental interest in Johnny behaving appropriately and doing well in school. I also challenged Johnny to name the parts of his father's concerns that might be valid. Johnny conceded that his grades were quite poor and that he would need to make changes in order to improve them. I validated Johnny for making what felt like a difficult acknowledgment. My underlying intention was to help Mr. Jones learn to acknowledge Johnny's improvements, no matter how small. I also wanted to help Johnny work more constructively with his father and find alternatives to acting out behavior. Literature on MDFT supports that the actualization of these treatment goals corresponds with reduced risk for adolescent substance abuse (Liddle et al., 2009; Henderson et al., 2010; Soderstrum et al., 2009).

Nevertheless, Johnny and Mr. Jones each re-asserted their positions with rising intensity. I interrupted to ask Mrs. Jones and Katrina what they thought might be happening between the men in their family. Mrs. Jones shrugged hopelessly. Contemptuously, Katrina bellowed that both her foster father and brother were "jerks;" Mr. Jones for being cruel to Johnny and Johnny for being lazy and refusing to do the immodest tasks that were asked of him.

Discussion Question: *At this point in the case, has your alliance with any particular individual family member in Johnny's family shifted ? If so, in what way, and why do you suppose that the shift occurred?*

____

____

____

____

____

____

As the first family session ended, I was feeling angry at Mr. Jones for being so demanding of Johnny, almost forgetting that Mrs. Jones was even there, eager to scold Katrina for being so obnoxious, and identifying strongly with Johnny. This initial session with the Jones' family told me a lot about my own biases and what it might be like for Johnny to be in his family. I needed to figure out how best to use this information that that will be shown to be highly valuable later in the case.

Right away, I recognized that the Jones families' chronic conflict, lack of consistent and reliable structure, and negative interchanges could make it easy for me to get overwhelmed and therefore distracted from the families' most pressing issues. The most pressing was Johnny's risk for suicide, though I was also eager to gather more historical information from the family, assess Mrs. Jones' for depression, and build a stronger alliance with Mr. Jones. It was obvious by this point in our work that he held the power in the family.

The Beginning of the Family Therapy: Getting to Know Johnny

For the first 6 months, I alternated weekly sessions with Johnny individually and then the entire family. In his individual sessions, Johnny staunchly denied ever having wanted to commit suicide. Instead, he merely took a significant number of pills based on a motivation to become severely intoxicated. He used most his time in session to complain about Mr. Jones' unfair treatment of him. Johnny's primary concerns were that Mr. Jones demanded that he come straight from home school and was rarely allowed to spend time with his friends. Johnny was also forced to wear clothes that Mr. Jones selected for him, rather than his preferred gothic attire. His chores consisted of strenuous yard work and auto detailing. As a punishment for unruly behavior, Mr. Jones would sometimes cut Johnny's hair despite lacking formal barber training.

Discussion Question: *What are your hypotheses' about Mr. Jones' parenting behavior? Assuming his good intentions, what might he by trying to accomplish and how could you use this re-frame in family therapy sessions to help the Jones family resolve conflicts?*

____

____

____

____

____

Johnny often reported feeling outraged. In response, I would empathize and listen supportively. When Johnny experienced intermittent calm and seemed more receptive to intervention, I would sometimes reflect that he was in no position to ask Mr. Jones for differential treatment due to his chronically poor grades and behavior. I reinforced that an adolescents' main priority should be to get good grades and stay out of trouble. In effort to inspire Johnny to be hopeful, I elaborated that, if Johnny were to improve his grades and behavior, I would advocate to Mr. Jones on his behalf. My intention was to delicately acknowledge the unreasonable nature of Mr. Jones rules and punishments, though to also challenge Johnny to do his part to earn privileges. I also thought this would provide a viable alternative to Johnny using his fathers' poor parenting to justify academic failure and acting out behavior. Ruiz et al.(2007) noted that these latter two negative outcomes are primary risk factors for adolescent substance abuse.

In family sessions that followed, I would often validate Johnny's feelings about being treated unfairly and then challenge him to reflect on the self-defeating nature of his efforts to retaliate against Mr. Jones. The latter intervention was put forth in front of Mr. Jones so as to build an alliance with him and to help Johnny consider more functional behavior. Connell et al. (2007) noted that decreases in adolescent conduct problems associate with decreased mental health symptoms. Both Johnny and Mr. Jones nodded affirmatively in response to my re-frame. I sensed that they both had at least an intellectual grasp of what I was saying, though neither was prepared to be the first to make important changes. Instead, each was waiting on the other to make the first concession.

In response to this stalemate, I proposed that, if Johnny presented weekly report cards that documented passing grades, I would be willing to meet with his *parents* and discuss potential rewards. I wanted to reinforce that *both parents together* should be making decision concerning Johnny and that Johnny's primary responsibility was to get good grades. It was important that I intervene on Johnny's behalf in ways that were respectful of the parental hierarchy. Research supports that this helps to maintain parental engagement in family therapy (Flicker et al., 2008). Johnny and Mr. Jones reluctantly agreed to my proposition. Katrina and Mrs. Jones did not respond verbally, though seemed to at least passively support anything that might decrease what seemed to be pervasive disagreement and family conflict. I was encouraged to see that there was some degree of consensus among all four family members. It is also important to note that my last intervention targeted all four domains in MDFT and it had a positive effect on the larger Jones family system. This positive result supports the theories' efficacy in practice.

The Beginning-Middle of the Jones' Families Therapy: Treatment for the Mothers

Approximately six months into therapy, the family members seemed more engaged. Each member told me more about his her perspective on what was happening in the family and about their lives as individuals.

In sessions with all family members present, Mr. Jones shared a deeper, underlying feeling of incompetence as a parent. Mrs. Jones disclosed that she often felt as if she wanted to take a long vacation and never come back. Katrina revealed a chronic feeling of hopelessness about her future. In response to each statement, there was a therapeutic silence. I allowed this silence because it seemed to allow each family member to have a healthy period of introspection that might lead to problem solving.

One month later, in an individual therapy session, Johnny reported that he "drank occasionally" with friends between classes. I encouraged him to tell me more about his drinking. Johnny defensively answered that he drank only when his friends supplied alcohol, which occurred "every so often."

Discussion Question: *Johnny's disclosure of abusing alcohol presents an ethical dilemma. As he is a minor, his parents would feel entitled to be informed, though informing them of his report would likely damage the therapeutic alliance with Johnny. How would you handle this and what would be the pros and cons of your decision?*

____

____

____

____

____

____

Rather than informing Johnny's parents, I decided to continue assessing Johnny individually. I hypothesized that Johnny might be testing whether or not I was trustworthy and that informing his parents of his drinking would lead Johnny to disengage from the therapy. Up to that point, Johnny's engagement had progressively increased. I also considered that his parents seemed to lack the parenting skills that would be necessary to intervene in Johnny's drinking in ways that would lead to a positive result.

Meanwhile, Katrina was making it known that her family members' ongoing conflicts were fast becoming intolerable to her. In session, she regularly threatened suicide. I referred her to the emergency room on five separate occasions. She repeatedly stated that she felt hopeless about her future and enraged at Mr. Jones and her brother for "making my life terrible." I tended to listen supportively and try to re-assure her that the family would continue to work on improving communication and that individual therapy for her would help her cope. My hope was that my empathic statements and her intermittent regulation in response would provide modeling for Mr. and Mrs. Jones. Typically, when Katrina would begin yelling and making threats, both parents seemed to become overwhelmed, afraid, and frozen.

Through extensive collateral work, I was able to secure a medication evaluation and individual therapy for Katrina. Within two weeks, she was markedly more stable and less emotionally reactive to Johnny and Mr. Jones' negative interchanges. As Katrina stabilized, I began to take more notice of Mrs. Jones' depressive presentation. Katrina's acting out responses to Mr. Jones' and Johnny's' conflicts may have been her best effort to provide the family with mothering given Mrs. Jones' incapacity. My hope was that helping Mrs. Jones get treatment for her depression might help her be a more active mother, shift the balance of parental power, and help Katrina return to a more developmentally appropriate role in the family.

Toward the end of a session when Mrs. Jones was noticeably more sad and lethargic, I reflected that she seemed to "have a lot on her plate." I then inquired about whether she might be interested in meeting with me individually. She readily agreed.

We met twice over the next month. When we met, Mrs. Jones' surprised me by speaking continuously for nearly the entire session. It felt as if she was unloading a century of pent up emotions. I learned that she was very angry about her family members' ongoing conflicts and suffering no matter what she did. This resulting feeling of failure led her to consider abandoning her family in the middle of the night.

Nervously, I asked her if she thought that she might be depressed. She agreed that she probably was. She also agreed to seek treatment. I provided her with a phone number to a local psychiatrist and encouraged her to set up an appointment at her earliest convenience. Within three – four weeks, her affect was noticeably brighter. Her family members shared a worry about how she was "always getting mad." I reflected that it might be good for her mental health to express her feelings. Burstein et al. (2006) noted that internalizing problems (i.e. what may have increased Mrs. Jones' vulnerability to depression) is a risk factor for destabilization within families affected by substance abuse.

The Middle of the Family Therapy: The Truth about Johnny Comes Out

After Mrs. Jones and Katrina began their individual therapies, the family as a whole began to show some signs of improvement. Johnny and his father's more serious arguments occurred less frequently. Katrina had not threatened suicide for two continuous months. These improvements are consistent with the predictions that MDFT produces results because it affects all members of the family system.

Soon after I began to appreciate the families' gains, Johnny presented to individual therapy with dilated pupils, profuse sweating, and a pale color to his skin. He was hyper, euphoric, and restless, which are key indicators of stimulant abuse (Ruiz et al., 2007). Given y working knowledge of substance abuse symptomology, I asked Johnny directly if he was intoxicated. He initially reported that he was not, though also asked if I would inform Mr. Jones of a potential disclosure. Hesitantly, I informed Johnny that whether or not I would talk to Mr. Jones about what I heard would depend on what Johnny told me. I let him know that a report of getting high every day and committing crimes to fund his substance abuse would have to be relayed to his foster parents, so as to ensure his livelihood. I added that irregular, recreational drug use need not be relayed to his foster parents. However, we would need to discuss his substance abuse and work towards decreasing it. I was transparent with Johnny so as to provide him with the information he needed to make his own decision. This general framework of working with ambivalence is consistent with motivational interviewing, an evidence-based approach to treating substance abuse (Ruiz et al., 2007). I also assured Johnny that I wanted to help him build a better life and was powerless to help him if he could not be honest with me. After some internal deliberation, Johnny admitted that he was high on methamphetamine. He added that his foster parents lacked the working knowledge of drugs to know that he was using, and pleaded with me to keep his secret. Facing quite the ethical dilemma, I called Mr. and Mrs. Jones and had them pick Johnny up early from therapy, as additional interventions would not be effective while he was intoxicated.

Discussion Question: *At this point in Johnny's treatment, what would you do and how would you handle his obviously increasing risk factors for substance abuse? What would be the pros and cons of your decision?*

____

____

____

____

____

Over the next week, I hypothesized that Johnny may have come to therapy in an intoxicated state as a cry for help. I also remained concerned about Mr. Jones highly concrete thinking, reactionary tendencies, and poor problem solving and parenting skills. This led me to wonder if informing him about Johnny's drug use would lead him to implement harsh and ineffective punishments, rather than helping him seek the substance abuse treatment services he obviously needed.

I therefore decided to meet with Johnny individually and construct our own substance abuse treatment plan. My thought was that Johnny would comply with the plan if compliance ensured that I would not tell his foster father about his drug abuse.

I called Mr. Jones and asked him to bring Johnny back for an individual therapy session the following week. When I met with Johnny, I let him know that I was very concerned about his substance abuse. I added that his problems in school and ongoing behavior problems were evidence that his substance abuse may have reached a level that required treatment.

Fearfully, Johnny protested. I assured him that I was not planning to tell Mr. Jones about his substance abuse as long as he was willing to develop a substance abuse treatment plan with me and bring evidence every week that he was complying with it. He readily agreed.

I informed him that he would be required to submit to random drug testing on same day notice and that our agency would provide the test kits. Johnny was also advised that he needed to produce weekly report cards that reflected passing grades in all classes. I added that passing grades would be evidence that he was in fact sober (as is often the case with teenagers in my experience). I added that any deviation from our agreement or failed drug tests would result in full disclosure of all incriminating circumstances. With wide eyes and shaking hands, Johnny agreed. As we ended the session, I invited Mr. and Mrs. Jones to enter my office from the lobby. I let them know that I was becoming increasingly worried about Johnny's poor grades and defiant behavior and therefore wanted to start randomly drug testing him. Mr. and Mrs. Jones readily agreed. The purpose of this intervention was to provide the benevolent parenting that and monitoring that would decrease Johnny's substance abuse, though also involve his parents to the greatest extent possible.

Over the next six weeks, Johnny passed three drug tests and his grades increased from F's into the D range. In individual therapy, Johnny talked to me about his efforts to avoid conflicts with Mr. Jones by isolating himself in his room. In family sessions, Mr. Jones denounced Johnny as being antisocial. In effort to reframe Johnny's best efforts at problem solving, I praised him for avoiding conflicts. Johnny seemed pleased with my reframe, though Mr. Jones was sullen and quiet.

Over the next month or so, Johnny came to therapy by himself or with Mrs. Jones. Katrina did not attend, though I was less concerned about this because I confirmed that she was attending her individual therapy and doing well. However, Mr. Jones' absence led me to wonder if I had become too allied with Johnny against Mr. Jones.

Meanwhile, Johnny's grades continued to improve. I sensed an age-appropriate incentive might help him capitalize on his recent momentum. I asked Mrs. Jones if she would allow Johnny to look into an internship at a skate board store, which he had previously talked to me about. Mrs. Jones agreed, and also agreed to discuss this plan with Mr. Jones. I was hoping that her inquiry would be a step in the direction of balancing the power in the parental unit.

Johnny and I enthusiastically began to set up interviews over the phone, which Mrs. Jones agreed to drive him to. Unfortunately, each interview was vetoed by Mr. Jones. Johnny would tell me at length about how this made him resentful. I internally agreed, though resisted my urge to collude with him. I was becoming increasingly certain that my imbalanced alliances with Mr. Jones and with Johnny associated with Mr. Jones' undermining of potentially helpful interventions. This association is consistent with the theories of family therapy that are discussed in Shelef et al. (2005). I was more fully realizing that interventions on Johnny's behalf would not be effective unless Mr. Jones and I were working together.

Discussion Question: *Working more constructively with Mr. Jones is now a more obvious necessity. What would you do, at this point, to build an alliance with him?*

The Middle-End of the Family Therapy: Getting to Know Mr. Jones

With great reluctance and overriding insistence from my clinical supervisor, I made a more heartfelt effort to engage Mr. Jones. After a month of unreturned phone calls, Mr. Jones called me back and requested that we meet privately. I agreed, and nervously confirmed in clinical supervision that he may have a grievance against me. I also concurred with my supervisor that I would need to hear, understand, and empathize with his concerns in order to re-engage him and thereby increase the positive potential of the therapy.

When Mr. Jones and I met, he indirectly informed me that he felt that he should have been more involved in important decisions pertaining to his son. His aforementioned disengagement and explanation of why is predicted by the family therapy theories discussed Flicker et al. (2008).

With sincerity, I assured Mr. Jones my good intentions and acknowledged that I had also felt like we "were going in different directions." I also added that I felt encouraged by his willingness to meet individually and that I would look forward to an opportunity to work with him, as would be necessary to help Johnny improve his grades and behavior.

Mr. Jones then revealed that he felt unfairly blamed for "everything" by his foster children. He elaborated that he felt obligated and even compelled to be strict because there were sex traffickers in his family who had sold his (now adult) nieces, nephews, and one of his other foster children into sex slavery. He told me that he found out three years prior and did not know what to do. His shame and sorrow were immense.

I now wonder if Mr. Jones called me because he needed to tell someone what happened. He may have felt no longer able to keep his traumas secret, as I once remember feeling about my own traumas when I finally started talking. It may have even been our shared emotional wounding that drew him in to see me that day.

Based on intuition, I validated Mr. Jones for coming forward about what happened and asked him if he would come see me privately over the next couple weeks. My thought was that this conjoint work (that is an integral part of MDFT) would help Mr. Jones relieve pent up emotions and therefore become more capable of positive parenting.

Discussion Question: *Has your view of Mr. Jones changed since the inception of the case? If so, how has it changed? Is there a lesson to be learned from this?*

I had figured out in the beginning of therapy that Johnny needed to be acknowledged for his incremental successes. I also knew it would mean the most to him to hear of his successes from Mr. Jones. However, Mr. Jones held a deep-seated shame and incompetence that made it impossible for him to give Johnny what he needed. In a sense, Johnny and Mr. Jones both needed a benevolent father figure.

In the weeks that followed, Mr. Jones told me about his own experiences of life as a foster child. He told me that he was always alone and angry throughout his early life in group homes and temporary foster homes He shared that his own terrible experiences in the foster care system inspired him to take good care of foster children. His hopes and dreams for Johnny were for him to grow up to be well-mannered, responsible, and more successful than Mr. Jones himself ever was. At the appropriate time, I validated the positive parenting aspects of Mr. Jones's disclosures, though also challenged him to consider acknowledging Johnny's relatively marginal improvements, even when they seemed to be grossly outweighed by his chronic behavior problems. My hypothesis was that praise from Mr. Jones would build Johnny's self-esteem and thereby improve his grades and behavior, as would be consistent with the theory of MDFT.

USING THE ALLIANCE WITH MR. JONES TO HELP JOHNNY GROW

While Mr. Jones and I were meeting individually, I also met with Johnny individually. I encouraged him to try to earn desired privileges from Mr. Jones rather than feeling unjustifiably restricted and then rebelling by playing internet pornography at high volume and using vulgar language. I validated Johnny's anger as understandable, though also challenged him to consider that he might be ruining his life in order to get back at Mr. Jones.

While Johnny was thinking about the aforementioned possibility, I encouraged him to construct a proposal to Mr. Jones to increase his grades into the passing range in exchange for certain privileges. I cautioned Johnny that Mr. Jones had the authority to approve or deny Johnny's proposal, and that he should therefore construct a proposal with reasonable and proportional improvements and rewards. This intervention is consistent with MDFT theories about helping substance abusing adolescents develop alternatives to substance abuse and related behavior problems.

I requested that all four family members attend the next session so that they all had input to Johnny's proposal and related negotiations that were sure to ensue. I began by summarizing my last individual session with Johnny so as to discretely cue Mr. Jones about the parenting-related content of our last session in a way that respected his parental authority. An agreement between Johnny and Mr. Jones would be important because, as noted by Burstein et al. (2006) positive parenting behaviors in present day interactions can begin to compensate for past relationships between parental psychopathology, negative parenting, and children internalizing their problems; which were some of Johnny's most prominent risk factors for substance abuse.

I was surprised and impressed to hear Mr. Jones request that Johnny write out a contract that promised an 8pm curfew every Friday and Saturday night that Johnny produced a weekly report card with C's or better in all classes for the previous week of school. Johnny openly suspected that Mr. Jones would not keep to his end of the agreement. Before Mr. Jones could defend himself, I challenged Johnny to *first* fulfill his end of the agreement and then advocate for himself. All family members seemed relatively satisfied.

Amazingly, Johnny produced weekly report cards that averaged C's or better for three weeks in a row. One week, he received all B's and A's. He told me that his friends learned of his accomplishment and, while he was still seated in his desk, he was carried out of class and paraded through the hallway. After a brief pause, he reported: "I think I have some self-esteem now."

Nevertheless, Mr. Jones refused to extend Johnny's curfew. Instead, he permitted Johnny to see certain friends on a more limited basis and to get his hair cut in a legitimate barber shop. In support of her brother, Katrina moved out of her room and into the garage with her cat, her "new family that wasn't corrupt."

Discussion Question: *Put yourself in Mr. Jones' position. What legitimate reasons might he have had for rescinding on his promise to Johnny for more privileges? Consider the parental responsibilities that were discussed in the theory of multi-dimensional family therapy and recommendations for family-focused treatment for adolescent substance abusers.*

____

____

____

____

____

____

I initially felt exasperated with Mr. Jones, though I ascertained in clinical supervision that Mr. Jones may have a logical basis for his decision and had still made some concessions. Whereas he initially refused to allow Johnny *any* freedom to see any of friends outside of school, he had gradually extended his permissions. So as to help Johnny continue on his upward path, I reinforced Mr. Jones' concessions and validated his feelings of betrayal. My intention was to support Johnny's emotions and help him see that his foster father could be reasoned with. I also validated Johnny's newly demonstrated ability to abide by rules that he did not agree with and concurred with his position to move out when he turned 18 in a few months.

The End: Termination

After a year of family therapy, Mr. Jones informed me that the family would be moving out of the area. He explained that a rural area he learned about offered inexpensive property in a good neighborhood. He added that his wife seemed pleased, though Katrina was very upset about the move, which she expressed by moving out of the garage into the shed in the backyard.

Mr. Jones noted that Johnny was also sad, though was handling the news much better than expected. Mr. Jones told me that he and Johnny sat down and had a talk after school a few days prior. Johnny was informed about where the family was moving and why. Johnny acknowledged that he would miss his friends, though he could understand his foster father's reasoning and interest in making Mrs. Jones happy.

I praised Mr. Jones for his transparent, respectful way of approaching Johnny. I reflected that Johnny may have taken the news so well because Mr. Jones had communicated the bad news so well. I suggested to Mr. Jones that he praised Johnny for this, and was encouraged to hear that Mr. Jones already had. Mr. Jones and I also agreed that the family would seek clinical services in their new locality.

A month after the family moved, Mr. Jones called me and reported that Johnny had been suspended from school for physically fighting with another student while he was intoxicated. Mr. Jones elaborated that he desperately wanted to seek treatment services for Johnny as soon as possible, which I helped to facilitate.

Johnny's relapse was of course disappointing. I was also encouraged by Mr. Jones' non-non-punitive, problem solving response that demonstrated a marked improvement in his parenting behavior. My sense was that Mr. Jones was now more capable of being the good foster parent he always wanted to be.

Discussion

It is important to first emphasize that the Jones' family was affected by multiple layers of problems, including intergenerational attachment issues, depression, and chronic relational conflict. These problems are supported by research to be risk factors for adolescent substance abuse (Beach et al., 2010; Sodertstrom et al., 2009; Liddle et al., 2009; Chasin et al., 2006; Kilpatrick et al., 2000; Burstein et al., 2006). The families' most formidable problems were Mrs. Jones' depression, and Mr. Jones and Katrina's psychopathology, which increased Johnny's risk factors for substance abuse. In order for Johnny to improve, his family members' individual issues needed to be treated. This is consistent with the predictions of MDFT theory. I will now discuss the recurring themes, interventions, and outcomes in the Jones family's therapy.

Johnny's conduct problems and poor grades made him easy to *blame*, which was a primary survival strategy in this family. Primarily, Mr. Jones and Johnny blamed each other, while Mrs. Jones, Johnny, and Katrina blamed Mr. Jones through a covert alliance. Blame-externalization was a survival strategy in the sense that it functioned as an alternative to family members' *internalizing negative feelings*, which was noted to be a risk factor for: adolescent substance abuse, Mrs. Jones' depression, and Katrina's risk for suicide.

I focused treatment on the families' blaming behavior because it incited family conflict that increased Johnny's risk for substance abuse. Johnny's blaming of Mr. Jones was also his primary excuse for repeated failures. I attempted to help Johnny develop alternatives to blaming by helping him work constructively with Mr. Jones and working with Mr. Jones to ensure that Johnny's efforts were reciprocated.

When the family members blamed each other in session, I often attempted to reframe blameworthy behavior in terms of its healthy attributes. This was my intention when I re-framed Johnny's isolation in his room as conflict avoidance. This was also my intention when I challenged Johnny to improve his grades before self-advocating for privileges.

The blaming family members (mainly Mr. Jones) often resisted these re-frames, particularly in the first half of the family therapy when we did not yet have strong working alliances. I nevertheless persisted with these intervention in order to help the family members see that no one individual family member was solely responsible for dysfunctional family dynamics. I also hoped to help the family members see that they could each make adjustments *as individuals* that would collectively decrease family conflict. For Mrs. Jones and Katrina, this primarily meant getting the individual treatment they sorely needed. For Mr. Jones and Johnny, this meant improving their communication. As predicted by MDFT, the actualization of these treatment goals associated with Johnny's notable improvements in academic performance and self-reported self-esteem during the same time period in which he decreased his substance abuse and behavior problems, family conflict decreased, each individual family member improved in functioning, and the individual family members and I had relatively balanced alliances.

CONCLUSION

I have presented a family therapy case example of the benefits of an MDFT-informed treatment approach. I have also demonstrated the efficacy of this approach to treating a more severe case of adolescent substance abuse. In particular, Johnny's case illustrated the more difficult to quantify and yet profoundly important principles of building and repairing therapeutic alliances and maintaining balanced alliances with all family members, and using those alliances to help adolescent substance abusers achieve therapeutic gains. My hope is that this chapter has demonstrated the efficacy of MDFT in theory and in practice.

Chapter 8

The Evolution of Inpatient Psychiatric Care: From Oppressive to Empowering Approaches

Severe mental illnesses are prevalent, damaging, and frequently go untreated until they pose a significant risk of harm. Half of all college-age Americans have a history of psychiatric disorder (Stone et al., 2012). However, "less than half of all Americans with a clinically diagnosable mental illness will ever receive treatment" (Schnittker, 2003, p. 507). This may be a consequence of the low insight that can be considered a symptom of severe mental illness (Munetz et al., 2001). The association between severe mental illness, low insight into the illness, and low level of treatment adherence may offer an explanation for the low quality of life that is normal for this population (Swanson et al., 2003).

The aforementioned association may also offer a partial explanation for why mental illness makes up a considerable share of a growing national health burden (Schnittker, 2003). From 1992 to 2001, there were 53 million emergency mental health contacts (Zeller, 2010). In 2002, the 1% of the US population that had schizophrenia amounted to a total cost of $63billion (DiBonaventura et al., 2012). 10% of patient populations have been found to be associated with 80% of direct costs associated with severe psychiatric illnesses (Winkler et al., 2011).

When mental illness impairs judgment to the point of creating risk of dangerousness to self or others, involuntary hospitalization becomes a necessary measure of last resort *and* provides an opportunity for impaired individuals to receive treatment (Winkler et al., 2011; Earley, 2006) For example, when individuals are acutely suicidal or hear command voices that tell them to harm themselves or others, hospitalization followed by emergency medications frequently leads to immediate, observable symptom decreases (Zeller, 2010). Frequently, psychotic patients report that *the loss* of their symptoms makes them feel alone, unimportant, and "that a return to madness is a better option than a 'sane' but socially impoverished life where so many developmental milestones have been missed," (Deegan, 2007, p. 66). The resulting disengagement from treatment frequently results in major cognitive disruptions, mood disturbances, and increased risk of dangerousness to self or others, which necessitates hospitalization (Jarrett et al., 2008). After being discharged, patients often disengage even further from mental health services in spite of the mortality, torment, disability, poverty, and isolation they live with (Munetz et al., 2001; Townsend, 2009). This is an example of how recovery from negative treatment experiences may be more challenging than recovery from the illnesses themselves (Roe et al., 2009). It is also an example of how mental health services can work against consumers rather than with them (Allison, 2012). Famously stated by Mahatma Ghandi: "The true measure of any society can be found in how it treats its most vulnerable members."

When we attempt to define dangerousness and competence, we raise important legalistic questions about human rights and the extent of dangerousness that necessitates hospitalization (Usahacharoenporn, 2011). Answering these questions requires consideration of the constitutional principle of individual freedom and the government's duty to care for individuals who are unable to care for themselves (Tataru et al., 2009). Consumers often advocate for reductions in forced treatments while clinicians often advocate for increases in their power to compel (Olsen, 2003).

Monahan (1993) states that ethically appropriate hospitalization is based on informed, competent, and well-coordinated risk assessment. Earley (2006) defines risk assessment as the clinician's determination of what is real and what is not real in the patients' disclosures. Essentially, this determination is an operational definition of what amounts to a hazy line between patient competence and incompetence (Borgeat et al., 2004). This determination necessitates a judgment call about when to overturn patient self-determination and informed consent (Nace et al., 2007). Ethically, clinicians must make this judgment call in spite of the professions' chronic failure to predict dangerous behavior (Olsen, 2003). Assessing for hospitalization also creates a dual role and threatens therapeutic alliances (Olsen, 2003; Bryden et al., 2010). At a more basic level, these discussions require an inherently problematic definition of what constitutes health and what constitutes illness, which suggests a normalcy standard of behavior and judgment and abnormalizes symptoms that are extreme forms of baseline humanity (Pesze, 1975; Olsen, 2003). Therefore, the subject of involuntary confinement and treatment lies at an important intersection of medicine, law, ethics, politics, and criminal justice (Earley, 2006).

In recent history, involuntary admits have increased by 50% and are generally detained for longer periods of time (Hughes et al., 2009; Iverson et al., 2009). They also present with higher symptom severity upon admission and represent the most severe and chronic cases that have the poorest treatment prognoses' (Hugo, 1999; McRee et al., 2012; Hopko et al., 2002). In a sense, involuntary patients need professional help the most and yet benefit from help the least, a paradox which underscores the need for more research on this topic (Swanson et al., 2003).

Writing Assignment: *Consider what you read in prior chapters. What are some culturally specific reasons that severely mentally ill patients of color may disengage from psychiatric treatment? If you were meeting with such a patient, and sensed the presence of these barriers to engagement, what might you say to the patient in session?*

____

____

____

____

____

____

In the literature review that follows, I will begin with a legal-historical overview of involuntary confinement and treatment, as separate entities. This is important because legalities and history guide all involuntary clinical practice (Monahan, 1993). I will then present some information on alternatives to psychiatric hospitalization, how inpatient hospitalization occurs, and how treatment is provided in inpatient settings. This will establish an environment-context for my next sections on pros, cons, and patient experiences with involuntary confinement *and* treatment. I will present these latter sections as one entity, *involuntary care.* I am combining these concepts at this point in my paper due to frequent similarities in research findings. I will then conclude with discussions of vulnerable population considerations, including psychiatric medication adherence, and limitations of existing research.

HISTORY

In the mid-19th century in the United States, mental illness was viewed as a symptom of spiritual deviation and was addressed in ways that severely restricted human rights (Pesze, 1975; Mrad, 2009). Doctors had virtually unchecked authority to commit the mentally ill to large, filthy, and overcrowded asylums (Fennell et al., 2006). This authority came from the states' *parens patriae* (e.g. parent) powers to confine patients who were deemed incapable of acting in their best interests (Pesze, 1975). The author elaborated that psychiatry and mental health held very little prestige in professional communities due to unlawful confinements, ineffective and unreliable treatments such as lobotomies, and poor prognoses.

Toward the end of the 19th century, the psychoanalytic school and other progressive scientific thought helped to inspire legal advocacy for procedural safe guards that mimicked criminal justice procedures (Pesze, 1975). This included formal notification of hearings and patient rights to jury trials (Fennell et al., 2006). The authors summarized the next 60 to 70 years of history as going back and forth from advancing patients' rights to increasing the state's powers to institutionalize.

In the 1960's and 70's, the civil rights movement helped to bring abuses and violations of patient rights into greater public awareness (Fennell et al., 2006). Mrad (2009) noted multiple Supreme Court cases that increased due process rights for the mentally ill who were facing civil commitment. In *Humphrey v. Cole* in 1972, the Supreme Court disagreed with prior judicial opinions on commitment not being a deprivation of liberty. The court expanded trial rights of the mentally ill on the basis that civil commitment is in fact a *massive* curtailment of liberty. In *Jackson v. Indiana* in 1972, the Supreme Court established grounds for limiting the length of civil commitment for patients who were committed so that they would be restored to competency to stand trial. The court also determined that the nature and duration of commitment must relate to the purpose for which the individual was committed. In *O'Conner vs. Davidson in 1975*, the Supreme Court extended basic human rights to people with mental disabilities (Taube, 2013b). The courts ruled that mental illness alone cannot justify civil commitment, *dangerousness* must also be present, and individuals should not be confined if they are capable of surviving independently or with the help of responsible friends (Fennell et al., 2006). In *Addington v. Texas* (1979), the Supreme Court ruled that the state always has the burden of proving *dangerousness* or *grave disability* in commitment hearings

(Usahacharoenporn, 2011). This case also set a *clear and convincing* evidentiary standard for commitment hearings, meaning a 75% probability that the evidence established a factual basis for the state's case (Hopko et al., 2002).

After debating patient rights in matters of involuntary *confinement* for over 100 years, the courts began to more fully examine involuntary *treatment* considerations in the 1990's (Mrad, 2009). In the landmark case of *Harper* in 1990, the US Supreme Court ruled that states can forcibly medicate prison inmates who are gravely disabled or are dangerous to themselves or others (Reamer et al., 1990). The court also determined that an administrative proceeding (rather than a hearing with a jury) is sufficient to determine whether involuntary medication is necessary (Breneman, 2004). Justices avoided the larger issue of whether or not involuntary medication was constitutional because they wanted to minimize legal system involvement in psychiatric decision-making (Baecht, 2009). In cases that followed, the courts ruled that mentally ill prison inmates can be forcibly treated with anti-psychotics if they are dangerous to themselves or others and antipsychotics are substantially likely to reduce presenting risk factors (Breneman, 2004). The author also presents the case of *Riggins v. US* in 1992, in which the Supreme Court affirmed that the mentally ill facing criminal charges generally retain the right to refuse antipsychotic medications. The courts also determined that this right can be overturned by a *compelling governmental interest* in prosecuting *serious crimes*. Side effects of forced medications must also be unlikely to interfere with the patient-defendants' participation in the trial.

Baecht (2009) discussed the landmark case of *Sell v. US* in 2002-2003. Prior to *Sell,* criminal defendants could be involuntarily medicated if a hearing officer determined that they were a) incompetent to stand trial b) dangerous to themselves or others c) gravely disabled, *or* d) unable to function in the general prison population. In *Sell,* The Supreme Court ruled that criminal defendants can be involuntarily medicated in order to restore their competency to stand trial and ultimately be punished provided there are legitimate government interests at stake, forced medications are likely to restore competency, no less restrictive alternative is available, and the medications are medically appropriate (Pietz, 2009; Breneman, 2004).

Several major cases have been decided based on the precedents set in *Sell* (Baecht, 2009). The author discusses a multitude of perspectives on the various consequences of this case, including delays of treatment and newfound case law. *Sell* also narrowed the legal definitions of dangerousness, due process rights, governmental interests, serious crimes, and the *substantial likelihood of medication effects* that are necessary to involuntarily medicate defendants. The author elaborated that important governmental interests (in this context) were eventually defined as the prosecution of serious (i.e. violent) crimes. Substantial likelihood of positive medication-treatment effect was defined as 50-70% likelihood of patient improvement. Dangerousness has been defined as imminent threat of death or great bodily injury (Fanniff et al., 2010). The dangerousness criteria was also expanded to allow for the confinement of those who are *gravely disabled* (Usahacharoenporn, 2011). This is defined as a condition that a) is likely to deteriorate irreversibly without intervention b) leads to complete neglect of basic needs for food, shelter, or personal safety, or c) leads to abnormal distress associated with the condition (Olsen, 2003).

In the 21st century, courts in Alaska set important precedents for patient rights in grave disability hearings (Breneman, 2004). Several of these precedents are reviewed by Usahacharoenporn (2011). In *Wetherhorn v. Alaska Psychiatric Institute* (2007), the court ruled that involuntary commitment of the gravely disabled requires that the individual be "incapable of surviving safely in freedom" (p.6). In *EP vs. Alaska* in 2008, the US Supreme court further interpreted the precedent-standards for civil commitment, ruling that it was unconstitutional to civilly commit a chronic gasoline inhaler on the grounds that he was dangerous to himself. The courts elaborated that the burden of proof lies with the state to show that the individual cannot take care of him or herself and that commitment is necessary to prevent the mentally ill person from severely and imminently harming him or herself or others. It was also clarified that socially unacceptable or unattractive behavior and mental illness, in and of themselves, are not enough to meet the requisite standard of proof for civil commitment. This argument forms the basis of a social psychological critique of grave disability (Catalano et al., 2007).

Writing Assignment: I*t has been established that clinicians are required to contact emergency service personnel when clients pose a significant risk of harm to themselves or others. A judgment call must be made about whether to inform the client about this contact being made. If you were meeting with an African American female who suffered from the delusion that her husband was having sex with staff members in her shelter, threatened to get a gun and kill him, and demanded that you maintain confidentiality, you would be legally required to contact law enforcement and the identified victim. Would you tell her that you were making these emergency contacts? Why or why not?*

____

____

____

____

____

____

INVOLUNTARY CONFINEMENT POLICY TO DATE

Salize et al. (2011) summarizes commitment reforms as generally attempting to reduce occurrences of involuntary commitment, though also aiming to protect mentally ill individuals themselves and society from dangerous manifestations of illnesses. Usahacharoenporn (2011) elaborates that courts hearing matters of commitment must balance the mentally ill's constitutional rights to liberty with the states' duties to provide care for the incapacitated and prevent harm in society. Taube (2013b) adds that this balance must be sought through the least restrictive treatment alternatives possible. The National Alliance on Mental Illness (NAMI), a consumer advocacy group, considers hospitalization the least restrictive alternative when severely mentally ill individuals are gravely disabled *and* likely to deteriorate without timely treatment, or lack the capacity to understand their need for care and make good judgments (Nace et al., 2007). This position that is generally consistent with the 5th standard of civil commitment in the state of Wisconsin (Spellecy, 2007).

Committed individuals must also have a mental illness and be gravely disabled or dangerous to themselves or others, though also have rights to appeal (Usahacharoenporn, 2011). Unlike criminal trials, commitment hearings do not require the petitioner to be competent, as the nature of confinement assumes some degree of incompetence which of course impairs the patient's ability to self-advocate (Fanniff et al., 2010). The authors elaborate that persons subject to civil commitment are afforded rights to counsel, call and cross examine witnesses, retain independent experts, and receive reasonable notification of hearings. The severely mentally ill are legally presumed competent to make treatment decisions in non-emergencies until proven incompetent by clear and convincing evidence (Munetz et al., 2001). This standard, in combination with the requisite relationship between reason for commitment and length and type of commitment, helps to ensure that only those who need to be committed are committed (Usahacharoenporn, 2011). In California, civil commitment policy ensures a formal review within the initial 72 hour 5150 hold period and then again within a 14 day 5250 hold period (Bernstein, 1988). In many jurisdictions, longer term commitments are reviewed every six to 12 months (Usahacharoenporn, 2011).

Taube (2013b) discusses the rights of confined patients. Patients have the right to not be unduly: restrained, isolated, medicated, abused, or neglected. Patients also retain rights to become educated, practice religion, engage in exercise and recreation, and refuse convulsive treatment for psychosurgery. The author elaborates that patient rights that may only be denied for good cause include the rights to confidentiality, wear their own clothes, have and use personal possessions, see visitors every day, have reasonable access to phones and letter writing materials, and to receive unopened correspondence. Such rights can only be denied if the exercise of those rights poses a legitimate risk of harm.

Usahacharoenporn (2011) notes that patients must be hospitalized at treating facilities of their choice and with providers of their choice, within the limits of available resources. Patients must also be hospitalized for the purposes of treating their condition, as evidenced by the construction of a treatment plan within 10 days of confinement (Bernstein, 1988). The author elaborates that the treatment plan must include goals, objectives, measures of progress, and periods of internal review. Treatment plans for involuntarily committed, gravely disabled individuals must target the symptoms of their grave disability.

President Jimmy Carter's vision of vast networks of halfway houses, group homes, foster care facilities, private hospitals, and community mental health centers inspired the community mental health movements of the modern era (Usahacharoenporn, 2011). These movements attempted to de-institutionalize the mentally ill and provide a majority of their care in the community (Fennell et al., 2006). The authors summarize the hypothesis that intensive case management services would link severely mentally ill individuals to housing and the multitude of services they would normally be provided in hospitals. However, communities were not provided with the resources that were necessary to provide adequate treatment. This resulted in alarmingly high numbers of homeless and incarcerated mentally ill individuals.

Putnam (2006) describes these individuals as tragedies to de-institutionalization and an example of a larger societal priority shift away from patient health toward public safety. This shift pits mental health workers against civil rights advocates and forces judges and police officers to work with high numbers of individuals they are ill-equipped to help. The authors elaborate that the courts essentially end up writing treatment plans for the chronically mentally ill. Usually, these individuals only get a semblance of treatment when they are incarcerated in settings that prioritize their confinement. This is at odds with a recovery model of mental health that moves away from a patient-provider battle of wills toward collaboration, treatment, and alliance building (Guarda et al., 2007; Swanson et al., 2003). The latter authors note that a more collaborative approach helps to extend "the greater societal goal of patient self-determination in healthcare . . . more fully to persons with psychiatric illness" (p. 474). "To be effective, the treating team must win patient's cooperation over time and persuade them to change their behavior," (Guarda et al., 2007, p. 108). The absence of which renders the hospital no different from a prison (Usahacharoenporn, 2011).

INVOLUNTARY TREATMENT

Since the 1950's, the mental health field has progressed from a medical model of caring for the incapacitated to greater consideration of their treatment needs as individuals (Salize et al., 2011). The invention of anti-psychotic medications in the 1950's contributed to an emptying of inpatient wards and increased the credibility of mental health professionals (Pesze, 1975). The author also noted that the discreditation of religious explanations of mental illnesses helped to expand professional interest in individual counseling.

Until the late 1970's, little distinction was made between involuntary confinement and treatment (Salize et al., 2011). The authors note that policy advances in this era created distinctions that helped to increase patient participation in treatment decisions, though falling short of allowing patients to refuse treatment under any circumstance.

In the 1980's, official policy increased the autonomy of severely mentally ill patients' (Munetz et al., 2001). The authors elaborate that policy makers reviewed important cases of patients who were involuntarily medicated. Policy makers concluded that high numbers of formerly hospitalized individuals were showing longer term signs of progress toward recovery. This helped to increase the credibility of mental health treatment for the severely mentally ill. In *Youngberg v. Romeo* (1982), the courts provided legal-ethical guidelines for the usage of involuntary medications. Guidelines required treating physicians to a) explain benefits and risks of medication to patients b) determine patient risk of harm to self or others before involuntarily medicating c) determine that the patient's condition would not improve (quickly) without medication, and d) obtain the concurring opinion of the hospital medical director (Mrad, 2009).

Mrad (2009) describes court cases from 1983 – 1989 that established conditions under which mentally ill individuals may refuse medications. In *Rennie v. Klein* (1983), the U.S. Court of Appeals reviewed a case that questioned whether involuntary medication violated the constitution's prohibition against cruel and unusual punishment. The court refused to decide firmly either way, though expressed some dissenting opinion about how involuntary medication in non-emergencies was a violation of citizen's emerging rights to privacy. This opinion formed the basis for the ruling in *Rogers* (1983) whereby it was concluded that a) involuntary commitment alone does not assume patient incapacity to make treatment decisions b) patients retain rights to refuse medications in non-emergency situations c) patients retain the right to not be secluded except in emergencies, and d) patients can only be involuntarily medicated with antipsychotics in order to prevent profound and irreversible mental health damage and not to maintain order on inpatients units or facilitate other institutional objectives. These cases are reviewed further by Sindel (1991) and The American Journal of Law and Medicine (1984).

In *People v. Medina* (1985), The Supreme Court of Colorado ruled that patients who refuse antipsychotic medication have rights to a hearing in which the state must prove a) treatment is necessary to prevent deterioration in the patient's condition b) no less restrictive alternatives are available *and* c) emergency treatment is necessary to prevent immediate or irreversible harm to the patient or those who would be injured by the patient's actions (The American Journal of Law and Medicine, 1984). The courts intended to limit the state's ability to administer involuntary treatment and to protect the rights of individuals who were less able to protect themselves (The American Journal of Law and Medicine, 1985).

In *Riese v. St Mary's Hospital & Medical Center* (1989), the Supreme Court of California ruled on whether patients who are committed to mental hospitals can be involuntarily medicated absent a judicial determination of incompetence (American Psychological Association, 2013). The APA rendered a legal brief on the positive treatment effects of antipsychotic medications, as well as their substantial side effects, and patient rights to make treatment decisions. Based on this brief, the court upheld inpatients' rights to refuse antipsychotic medication except when a judge determines they are incompetent or to prevent immediate and irreversible harm.

From 1990 – present, official policy on the usage of involuntary medications has been further specified in important cases. Near the turn of the century, there was a lack of consensus about whether involuntary patients should retain the same rights to refuse treatment in non-emergencies that are generally retained by voluntary patients (Reamer et al., 1990). In *Weston* (2001), the Supreme Court affirmed that criminal defendants can be involuntarily medicated in order to restore their competency to stand trial as long as the side effects of the medication were unlikely to interfere with the defendant's exercise of rights in a fair trial (Mrad, 2009). In *Myers* v. *Alaska Psychiatric Institute* (2006), the courts ruled that patients cannot be involuntarily medicated unless the medication is determined to be in the patients' best interests and all less intrusive options have been exhausted (Usahacharoenporn, 2011). There has been a recent movement in the US toward ending the usage of involuntary treatments altogether, which was case studied at a well-known Massachusetts' child/adolescent hospital that profoundly decreased its usage of involuntary medications, mechanical restraints, and related costs (Lebel, 2007).

Involuntary Treatment Law and Ethics to Date

Involuntarily committed mentally ill patients generally retain rights of informed consent to make treatments decisions unless there is a court order to the contrary (Salize et al., 2011; Taube, 2013b). Informed consent permits refusal of psychiatric medications except in psychiatric emergencies, which are defined as imminent risk of patient harm to self or others (Olsen, 2003; Vuckovich et al., 2005; Bryden et al., 2010). Research supports that assault or threat of assault is the most common basis for involuntarily medicating patients (Jarrett et al., 2008). Patients may also be involuntarily medicated if they are deemed *gravely disabled*, as defined by incapability to make informed decisions concerning treatment and other important affairs (Munetz et al., 2001; Pietz, 2009). This definition extends the dangerousness criteria into an ethical justification for forced treatment (Olsen, 2003). Summarized by Jarrett et al. (2008), ". . . the association between mental disorder and risk that autonomy is over-ridden not just in cases where people *cannot*, but also where they *will not* consent to treatment" (p. 545).

The previous description of the dangerousness criteria also forms the basis of the code of ethics for The American Medical Association (Hartmann, 2009) and The American Nursing Association (Vuckovich et al., 2005). The AMA mandates that individual autonomy must be respected by practicing professionals, though irrational or impaired individuals are not considered autonomous. The ANA mandates that coercion should be avoided and patients should participate in decision making about their own care *to the maximum extent possible*. Regan (2010) further elaborates on the difficulty of resolving ethical dilemmas in health care settings. Difficulties may relate to differences in practitioner a) morality about right and wrong b) assessment of patient mental health c) treatment philosophy and preference, e) decision making occurring on multiple levels f) experience, training, and expertise, and g) accountability to various stake holders. The authors emphasize that these differences are particularly manifest when practitioners are deciding whether to utilize involuntary treatment mechanisms such as medications and restraints. This offers some support for Iverson et al.'s (2009) concerns about medical model-driven assessments of patient competency to make treatments decisions, as well as Jarrett et al.'s (2008) recommendation for additional staff training in de-escalation strategies that may help to minimize the usage of coercive tactics.

Vuckovich et al. (2005) discusses California law on the subject. When patients and treatment providers disagree about whether medications are needed, patients may request capacity hearings. These occur infrequently and only after the initial 72 hour hold has expired and a 14 day extended hold has been upheld in a probable cause hearing. Patient and interested-party testimony, patient advocate persuasion, nurse incident documentation, and psychiatrist testimony are weighed in a judicial process of deciding whether or not a patient is competent to make treatment decisions. Within 72 hours, decisions about patient competency can be appealed through a writ hearing in probate court, though patients must take medications until that hearing.

Writing Assignment: *What are your beliefs and opinions about involuntary confinement and treatment? Are these beliefs and opinions more or less consistent with the way you usually relate to authority figures? How might these beliefs and opinions help to facilitate your clinical work with populations that often have difficulty negotiating relationships with authority figures, such as chronically homeless populations or children and adolescents? How might these beliefs and opinions be liabilities with these populations?*

____

____

____

____

____

____

ALTERNATIVES TO INSTITUTIONALIZATION

Advanced directives, involuntary outpatient commitment, and private hospitalization are alternatives to involuntary public inpatient hospitalization. Spellecy (2007) conceptualizes the initial two alternatives on a continuum of less restrictive alternatives to inpatient care. These alternatives help to prevent harm and restore patient *autonomy*, a core concept in the larger subject matter. Privatization will be shown to be a growing trend in psychiatric care that has important implications for the future of emergency mental health.

Advance Directives

Recently, there has been more usage of advanced directives for mentally ill patients who become unable to make important decisions and want decisions to be made for them based on what they would have wanted when of sound mind (Mental Health Weekly, 1999; Borgeat et al., 2004). The directive can be used to override patient treatment refusals that are expressed in a non-sound state of mind (Spellecy, 2007). The author notes that advanced directives for the mentally ill are now recognized in 25 states in the US. They are also used in many foreign countries (Salize et al., 2011).

Henderson et al. (2007) studied the effects of advanced directives and note that they significantly reduce violence, self-harm, and the need for involuntary care. Based on research outcomes, the authors recommend that advance directives include input from the patient, family members, and the treatment team. The authors elaborate that the directive should comprehensively identify the nature of presenting illnesses, warning signs for relapse, and preferred treatments in periods of incapacity.

There should be differences in advanced directives for intermittently competent mental patients and for the more seriously incapacitated patients (Munetz et al., 2001). The intermittently competent should appoint their own decision maker by proxy, who would be instructed by the patient about how decisions should be made in periods of incapacitation (Borgeat et al., 2004). The authors also elaborate on advance directives for more chronic, incapacitated individuals. In such cases, it may be necessary to court-appoint a conservator or limited guardian. Ideally, the guardian should only make decisions for the incapacitated individual in matters that the individual cannot reasonably make good judgments about, such as medical treatment. Guardians may be provided by a local nonprofit agency, which relieves family members of the burden of care. Guardianship also provides the mentally ill individual with an advocate with first-hand knowledge of the condition and possibly even personal experience with mental illness. The latter factor may help to increase adherence with treatment and alleviate the concerns of patient rights advocates.

Involuntary Outpatient Commitment (IOP)

Outpatient commitment has been gaining popularity in the United States in spite of controversy related to infringements on civil liberties and the extension of unwanted social control into vulnerable communities (Fennell et al., 2006; Putnam, 2006; Swanson et al.,

2003). The latter authors recount the advancement of involuntary outpatient commitment with the passage of Kendra's Law in New York in 1999. This law was passed in response to multiple innocent bystanders being pushed in front of subways by untreated mentally ill individuals. This law allows for the involuntary inpatient confinement of mentally ill individuals who do not adhere to their outpatient treatment plan, which may include psychiatric medications. Proponents claim that outpatient commitment provides an incentive to for patients to avoid re-hospitalization, improves adherence with medication and other treatments, and improves the continuum of care between inpatient and outpatient facilities, which helps to improve patient quality of life after discharge.

Research supports the overall efficacy of involuntary outpatient commitment (Spellecy, 2007). It has been found to reduce inpatient hospitalizations, lengths of inpatient stay, arrests, and risk of violence (Nace et al., 2007; Swanson et al., 2003). The latter authors conclude that IOP enables more consistent adherence to treatment by paradoxically detracting from patient autonomy in order to advance it. Nace et al. (2007) similarly discusses swift and predictable punishments as psychologically powerful motivators to positively change patient behavior. This theory has been corroborated in involuntary studies of: drug courts and addiction treatment, sports psychology, gender-specific issues, and disability benefit hearings. The authors conclude that the long term benefits of IOP, therefore, outweigh the shorter term disadvantages provided that involuntary orders are sustained and carried out by committed and response clinicians. Swanson et al. (2003) takes this last point a step further in arguing that re-hospitalization of involuntary outpatients may suggest that providers are committed to patient recovery.

Privatization

The privatization of psychiatric hospitals is a subject of considerable ethical debate (Beaulaurier, 2001). The author notes that privatization saves public dollars and is often argued to increase efficiency of treatment based on the theory that private companies will compete for government contracts. This is a dehumanizing way to talk about human suffering that is nevertheless necessary in light of scarce public resources (Hugo, 1999).

Beaulaurier (2001) reports that the primary argument in disfavor to privatization is that the quality of care will go down, which is not supported by evidence from practice. The author and Hugo (1999) note recurrent, mixed efficiency and outcome ratings for public and private facilities. It is also important to mention that public hospitals often admit involuntary patients that are deemed too severe and/or violent for private hospitals, which could skew outcome data (Stellwagen et al., 2010). It is therefore possible that there is a relative discrepancy in the quality of public-private inpatient psychiatric care, though further study is needed to establish a stronger research basis for the aforementioned arguments for and against.

INTERNATIONAL

It is important to discuss international research on involuntary care so as to comparatively analyze regional differences in laws, policies, procedures, and research data collection practices and findings (Georgieva et al., 2012; Salize et al., 2011). Fennell et al. (2006) summarizes Great Britain's long history of confining the mentally ill for more politically conservative reasons. Unlike the United States, Great Britain has never required dangerousness to be present. Confinement is usually authorized when it is presumed to be in the patient's best-interests and necessary to protect society from antisocial behavior.

Policy advances in Great Britain in the 19th century helped to reduce the frequency of arbitrary and unnecessary confinement. In Nottage v. Ripley (1849), the British Commission on Lunacy ruled that the mentally ill could be detained on *Parens Patriae* grounds, though relatives could block the detention by agreeing to care for them. In response to wrongful conviction scandals, The Lunacy Act of 1890 required that committed individuals be judicially certified and for the purposes of treating their illnesses.

In the 20th century, British policy helped to reduce stigma associated with mental illness and expanded patient rights to receive treatment (Fennell et al., 2006). The Mental Deficiency Act of 1913 authorized commitment of personality disordered individuals who could benefit from treatment. The Mental Treatment Act of 1930 brought policy more in line with the practices of medicine (and away from criminal justice policy) by allowing voluntary patients to be admitted through an interview with the hospital manager. Previously, voluntary patients had to go through formal court proceedings. The Mental Health Act of 1959 mandated the construction of mental hospitals that were strictly for the mentally ill who were committed because they were determined to be dangerous. The Act also decreased stigma by allowing treatment without certification of lunacy and authorizing health tribunals to review patient's needs for ongoing, involuntary detention.

In the 1980's, policy advances in Great Britain discouraged confinement and promoted access to treatment (Fennell et al., 2006). Hughes et al. (2009) discusses the landmark Mental Health Act of 1983, which was intended to expand the availability of psychiatric intervention for severely mentally ill individuals

Fennell et al. (2006) elaborated on various cases that lead to expansion of the usage of conditional release from involuntary inpatient care via community treatments orders. These orders clarified the terms under which patients could live in the community, provided they complied with their care plan. Unfortunately, health officials responded by increasing admissions of patients they had no plan to provide real treatment for. This practice was addressed and subsequently outlawed by the judiciary in the case of R. vs. Hallstrom (1985). The courts ruled that re-admission to the hospital due to non-compliance with the community treatment order required that the patient receive treatment for his or her primary mental condition. The Court of Appeals clarified that the Mental Health Act does not permit involuntary *treatment* (i.e. involuntary medication) of patients who are not detained in hospitals, nor does it prohibit patients from seeking judicial review of their confinement order (The British Medical Journal, 1986).

Fennell et al. (2006) also discussed British cases from the turn of the 20th century cases that further clarified the scope of community treatment orders. The Patients in Community Act of 1995 expanded the definition of treatment orders to include a supervised discharge plan. Patients who were dangerous to themselves or others *or were at serious risk of being exploited* could be mandated to live in a specific supervised place of residence in the community. They could also be required to participate in education or vocational training services. In DR v. Merseycare (2002), the government ruled that patients in supervised after-care cannot be required to take medications unless they are detained based on application of the principles of the Mental Health Act of 1983.

Over the last decade, the trend in public concern in Great Britain has been in the direction of protecting society from violent mentally ill individuals (Hughes et al., 2009). This inspired passage of the Mental Health Act of 2007, which expanded the criteria for involuntary detention, and more conservatively authorized it by expanding the definition of what constitutes a mental disorder and which professional disciplines that can be involved in treatment decision-making. Recent British policy advances have made it easier to involuntarily confine and treat patients who are generally considered treatment-resistant (Jarrett et al., 2008).

Community Treatment Orders (CTOs) have also become more popular in Australia (Segal et al., 2008). The authors elaborated that CTO's were introduced as a less restrictive alternative to involuntary hospitalization for patients who were decompensating in community living. CTO's were also used as discharge plans. More conservatively than in Great Britain, Australian mental patients detained under CTO's are not only required to live in a particular location, but they must also take prescribed medications, attend counseling, and abstain from illicit substances. The authors studied the efficacy of involuntary outpatient commitments in Australia and concluded that they help to reduce inpatient admissions and lengths of stay. Australia also requires extensive professional review of commitments in order to establish ongoing medical necessity (Xiao et al., 2004). Official policy discourages involuntary treatments such as mechanical and or physical restraints, seclusion, forced medications, and restrictions on leaving inpatient units (Ancstis et al., 2013).

Industrialized European countries made important advances in patient rights. Over time, policy in Scandinavian countries has generally progressed towards discouraging involuntarily confinement, compulsory medication, banning outside visitation, seclusion, and taking patients' property into official custody (Iverson e et al., 2009; Rydelius, 2007). Italian reforms have established restrictions on the usage of involuntary treatment mechanisms, which can only be authorized by physicians are considered measures of last resort (Del Vecchio et al., 2010). Italian laws also discourage institutionalization through advancing community care options (Girolamo et al., 2008). The authors elaborate that involuntary admission is only permitted in cases where intervention is a) necessary b) refused c) not possible to implement on an outpatient basis d) authorized by two physicians and the city mayor, and is subject to review in court.

China passed its first national health law in 2012 in response to growing concerns about the economy and related impacts on common citizens' quality of life (Phillips et al., 2013). The authors elaborate that the law shifted the focus of service delivery from specialized psychiatric hospitals to general hospitals and community clinics. In another paper, Phillips (2013) describes the health law as promoting de-institutionalization in similar fashion to the Western countries that were discussed previously.

Providing Treatment

Now that I have discussed the laws pertaining to involuntary confinement and treatment, I will present information on inpatient hospital settings and treatment procedures. This will include best practices for avoiding usage of coercive tactics, and how to incorporate patient-centered strategies when coercive tactics must be used (Zeller, 2010). As discussed previously, this is necessary because involuntary admits are frequently the most acutely mentally ill patients whose conditions predispose them to dangerous behavior (Pesze, 1975; Spellecy, 2007; Usahacharaoenporn, 2011). Coercion may be justified a) on the grounds of *beneficence*, or to do good b) after failed negotiations with patients, c) when psychosis overrides the therapeutic effects of a working alliance d) when untreated symptoms maintain ongoing patient suffering e) when medications are refused and are vital to patient recovery, and/or f) when patients are dangerous to themselves, other patients, or staff (Vuckovich et al., 2005; Anestis et al., 2013).

Coercive tactics may be necessary in the short term, though counterproductive in the long term in so far as creating antipathy towards providers and treatment itself (Stellwagen et al., 2010; Anestis et al., 2013; Swanson et al., 2003). Therefore, the decision to use coercive tactics and the particular tactic chosen should be proportional to the severity of threat to the patient and likelihood that treatment will be beneficial (Olsen, 2003; Georgieva et al., 2012). Guarda et al. (2007) frames this as a balance of safety and therapeutic factors (Guarda et al., 2007). The complexity of this dilemma necessitates some discussion of psychiatric hospital settings and protocols. This discussion will help to provide a context for my discussion of best practices.

Inpatient Hospital Settings and Protocols

Zeller (2010) notes that inpatient psychiatric hospitals generally have a particular design, structure, and protocol that is designed to maximize treatment efficiency and efficacy. Treatment may be provided a) through a psychiatric consultant seeing patients in a medical setting b) a psychiatric department in an emergency medical setting, or c) a stand-alone Psychiatric Emergency Services (PES) facility that only treats acute psychiatric patients. It is first necessary to determine whether patients have co-occurring medical etiologies, which is common in inpatient psychiatric settings (Zeller, 2010). Providers must then differentiate delirium from psychosis, as prescribing treatment for the former condition as if it were the latter can be life threatening. Treatment primarily consists of medications and counseling. Patients also require a sufficient number of qualified nursing staff, vital sign monitoring, behavioral observation, critical nursing care, and video recording to monitor usage of involuntary treatments (Winkler et al., 2011; Anestis et al., 2013).

According to the US Surgeon General: "Mental health care occurs relatively frequently in emergency rooms and psychiatric hospitals. These settings and patterns of treatment undermine the delivery of high-quality mental health care" (Catalono et al., 2007, p. 89). Patients with acute disturbances of thought, mood, or behavior are frequently provided services in under resourced psychiatric settings (Pesze, 1975). Providers must admit the patient or rapidly stabilize them and refer them out (Zeller, 2010). Admission numbers may vary on the basis of inpatient bed space and the treatment philosophy of psychiatrists and other mental health professionals (Girolamo et al. 2008). The average length of stay in inpatient psychiatric hospitals is generally declining (Fanniff et al., 2010). Unfortunately, this may have less to do with improved patient outcomes and more to do with managed care emphasis on cost containment (Lyons et al., 1997). Patients usually receive an intake by one professional, are care managed by a team, and are triaged by another professional who makes decisions concerning their disposition (Monahan, 1993). The author elaborates that the ultimate decision maker is likely to be an overburdened professional who does not have the time to read voluminous patient chart information and might therefore make a hasty decision based on limited acquired information. Olsen (2003) adds that inpatient professionals frequently lack the intimate knowledge of the patient that individual therapists may have. This lack of information can make it particularly difficult to determine whether involuntary hospitalization is necessary.

Coercive tactics may be necessary in order to facilitate important aspects of hospital programming (Stellwagen et al., 2010). The author describes the two primary coercive tactics, seclusion and restraint. Seclusion is the isolation of a patient in what is often a padded room. Restraints are mechanical devices (or straps) that are used to restrict patient movement. These devices make it possible to involuntarily medicate patients who are highly aggressive (Winkler et al., 2012). Olsen (2003) adds that many of patients' rights are restricted in inpatient care, including a) patients' decisions of daily life, e.g. what food they can eat b) meaningful activities, e.g. access to work, c) choice of treatment, d) control of resources, e.g. money), and e) emotional or verbal expression. Interestingly, research supports that increased usage of involuntary treatments *and* strong, official discouragement of usage of involuntary treatments associate with higher rates of inpatient violence (Steinert, 2007; Rydelius, 2007).

Psychiatric Nursing Approaches to Inpatient Care

Frequently, nurses frequently have the most contact with psychiatric patients (Vuckovich et al., 2005). The authors note that they must always strive to balance the ethical principle of beneficence with the duty to respect patient autonomy throughout all aspects of daily hospital programming. An individualized approach is necessary to determine what will be most effective and least harmful for the patient (Georgieva et al., 2012). This is an empathic knowledge, sensitivity, and flexibility that surveyed patients advise treatment professionals to acquire (Bentley, 2010). It also coincides with increasing official recognition that patients should be more involved in their own health care (Dyck et al., 2005). An individualized, empathic approach is particularly necessary for psychotic patients who may have difficulty expressing their needs and lack the insight that is necessary to make autonomous decisions (Andreasson et al., 2012; Spellecy, 2007). For similar reasons, Guarda et al. (2007) goes so far as to call it arrogant to treat all patients equally, particularly *professional patients* who frequent inpatient hospitals and treatment centers. Orienting treatment to individual patient perspectives and experiences is essential to “the ideal of a therapeutic alliance . . . that all mental health professionals aspire to” (Morrison et al., 2000, p. 815). Alliance ultimately predicts patient adherence to treatment plans and results in positive behavior change (Schnittker, 2003).

Nurses are often very good at convincing patients to take their medications, as evidenced by the relatively significant difference between total involuntary admits and number of capacity hearings to determine if medications can be given involuntarily (Vuckovich et al., 2005). The authors qualitatively interviewed nurses who reported that they infrequently have to strap patients down and involuntarily medicate them after the first couple days of hospitalization. The authors consider this encouraging because patient consent to oral medication reduces the negative effects of coercion. Oral consent is also generally as effective as intramuscular formulation (Georgieva et al., 2012). These reports of nurses facilitating medication adherence may offer some support for the increasing trend of nurses prescribing, administering, and monitoring-managing psychiatric medications (Allison, 2012). Ethically, this practice requires that nurses have advanced technical knowledge of medications (Jones et al., 2007).

Nurses utilize a variety of therapeutic strategies to avoid coercion. They frequently attempt to avoid or at least prolong coercion by establishing rapport and mutual agreement on treatment plans, respond to patient resistance by advocating for changes of treatment plans, and more comprehensively and intuitively assess early stage patient escalation, which often leads to creative interventions (Regan, 2010; Vuckovich et al., 2005). The latter authors report that nurses frequently: advise patients that medications will improve their functioning, inform them of the positive consequences of adherence, and clarify the negative consequences of noncompliance, including the possibility of extended hospital stays. Nurses do not consider these statements threats, they consider it persuasion and frequently report a deep desire to avoid using coercive tactics (Deegan, 2007).

Vuckovich et al. (2005) describe nurses as frequently shying away from extensive negotiation with resistant patients. They usually back off when an impasse about taking medications is reached and medication refusal does not create a significant risk of harm. This approach is consistent with consumer recommendations for providers to be more patient and treat patients as dignified human beings (Bentley, 2010). Nurses frequently feel proud about having avoided the usage of coercive tactics and feeling a sense of failure when they must be used (Chiovitti, 2011; Regan, 2010; Vuckovich et al., 2005). The authors elaborate that nurses feel particularly distraught about involuntarily medicating patients who would never take medications voluntarily, regardless of symptom remission.

When coercion must occur, nurses yell “now” to signal their team, strap the patient down, and involuntarily medicate them (Vuckovich et al., 2005). The authors report that nurses frequently stay with patients afterwards in order to debrief, assure them that they will not be abandoned, and assure them that the intent was to help. This provides patients with opportunities to introspect about what happened and how future instances of compulsory treatment might be avoided (Andreasson et al., 2012). This debriefing strategy is consistent with Cohen’s (2012) noted moral duty of practitioners to protect consumers by scrutinizing clinical paradigms that reinforce professional power and behavioral expressions of it.

The aforementioned nursing strategies are consistent with the theory of *protective empowerment* described by Chiovitti (2011). According to this theory, patients should be allowed to make choices within the limits of their health and should generally retain their autonomy. Nurses can help patients achieve these goals through interactively teaching, encouraging patient health and wellness, maintaining safety, and avoiding power struggles. This theory parallels Zeller’s (2010) recommendations for a more integrated medical model of psychiatric care. He recommends that interventions should flow from a combination of the compassionate therapeutic approaches of psychiatry and the fast-paced assessment and treatment approaches of emergency medicine. These theories are supported by research findings that patient participation helps to facilitate recovery in even the more severe and chronic cases (Georgieva et al., 2012; Munetz et al., 2001; Bentley, 2010). The fairly recent development of these theories is consistent with the evolution of psychiatry from a frequently abusive, paternalistic model (that formed the basis of older objections to involuntary care) to a more patient-centered model of integrated rehabilitation (Pesze, 1975; Bentley, 2010).

Writing Assignment: *You are in a psychiatric inpatient settings and are working with a middle aged Caucasian woman who presents with symptoms of mania, including pressured speech, irritability, elevated energy, grandiosity, and several recent hospitalizations related to manic presentation. She also has a significant history of sexual and physical trauma. She is adamant that she does not have a mental health issue, has been unjustly hospitalized, and perceives herself as victimized by her confinement. Put yourself in her position. How is she feeling and why?*

____

____

____

____

____

____

Challenges to Avoiding Coercion

Stellwagen et al., (2012) recommends the critical analysis of factors that contribute to usage of involuntary treatment mechanisms. The authors elaborate that this will help to identify opportunities for preventative interventions. Chiovitti (2011) describes multiple factors that can lead to involuntary treatment administration, including patient: suicidal behavior, withdrawn psychotic symptoms, agitation, aggression, staff manipulation, and attention-seeking behavior. These patient factors may generate problematic emotional responses in inpatient staff, including helplessness, avoidance, withdrawal, guilt, fear, provocation, lack of control, anger, intolerance, powerlessness, over-protective tendencies, feeling drained, and inter-staff divisions. Related interplays may lead staff to overlook patient self-determination and impose unnecessary restraints or activity limitations. This may offer a more pragmatic explanation for what are historically condescending and even abusive positions taken on inpatient units (Pesze, 1975).

Therapeutic approaches help to decrease the likelihood that coercive interventions will be necessary in various instances. A motivational admission interview in the first staff-patient contact helps to establish that staff are empathic, though patients are ultimately responsible for changing their own behavior (Stellwagen et al., 2010). Throughout treatment, it is continuously necessary to give patients latitude to manage their behavior and also maintain some personal responsibility for their own safety (Chiovitti, 2011). The authors interviewed psychiatric nurses who reported that patients often suffer over what may be trivial affairs. Nurses acknowledge that they must nevertheless take patient concerns seriously, acknowledge them, and responded in ways that empower patients to feel adequate and capable. For example, teaching patients coping skills helps them divert from their symptoms and the possibility of extended hospitalization (Olsen, 2003). This can be a particularly empowering alternative for patients who are self-harm risks, who might otherwise have their movements restricted (Hughes et al., 2009).

Discharge Planning

Discharge planning is an integral part of inpatient care as it helps patients transition back into society (Andreasson et al., 2012). It can also be considered the start of a more full and authentic recovery (Hughes et al., 2009). Follow up care helps to prevent decompensation and re-hospitalization by providing additional supports that help patients manage symptoms (Townsend, 2012 ; Girolamo et al., 2008). Unfortunately, it is rare for inpatient facilities to follow up to ensure that discharge plans were followed through on (Monahan, 1993). This is of particular concern because more violent patients are often discharged to poor quality facilities that they quickly abandon and are then at increased risk for committing another act of violence (Pesze, 1975; Girolamo et al., 2008).

Girolamo et al. (2008) note that patient adherence to discharge plans can be improved by clearly stating the risks associated with treatment drop-out to both patients and their family members. Patients should also be better prepared for discharge when they are still in the hospital (Chiovitti, 2011). Such risk prevention planning is particularly necessary when discharging suicidal patients (Skeem et al., 2006). Encouragingly, these patients can often be quickly and safely discharged soon after admission (Zeller, 2010). The author notes that this is often true if a) the suicide attempt was a reaction to a precipitating event that the patient has acquired a new perspective on b) the plan and intent had low chances of lethality c) they have supportive and stable housing, and d) they are capable of and motivated to follow up with their discharge plan.

Family Involvement

Paradoxically, patient's family members are often centrally involved in their confinement and treatment as well as their recoveries (Usahacharoeporn, 2011; Andreasson et al., 2012). Severely mentally ill adults are often an extreme care burden to their family members who may have their own mental health issues and become overly emotionally involved in the care process (Bentley, 2010; Garcia et al., 2006; Girolamo et al. 2008). This may help to explain the high levels of family conflict that are noted by the latter authors to be typical of severely mentally ill populations. This may also explain why family conflict is the primary precipitant of psychiatric crisis and subsequent hospitalization that is usually initiated by family members involved in care (Girolamo et al., 2008; Camacho et al., 2012). Bentley (2010) elaborates that families are frequently frustrated by patient nonadherence, the limits of medications, and provider refusals to confine and treat (Earley, 2006). Family members often interpret these refusals as evidence that professionals are unconcerned (Borgeat et al., 2004).

Family involvement and support has been shown to improve outcomes for involuntary patients (Tolou-Shams et al., 2012; Bruns et al., 2012). Family members can help patients understand their need for professional help, maintain their identities during involuntary confinement, and maintain or improve psychiatric medication adherence (Hughes et al., 2009; Townsend, 2012). Families can also help to decrease patient access to street drugs that may compromise health and recovery, improve the overall course of psychiatric illness, and improve adherence to discharge plans (Garcia et al., 2006; Ebner et al., 2007). Family involvement tends to reduce unnecessary hospitalizations (Usahacharoenporn, 2011). A lack of family involvement predicts re-hospitalization (Camacho et al., 2012; Lyons et al., 1997).

Writing Assignment: *Why might the family members of severely mentally ill clients of color be reluctant to participate in their care? Consider that families of color often have practical limitations, though are also resilient and therefore adept at coming up with innovative solutions to overcome these barriers. Thus, practical limitations are often stated to providers, though may also mask deeper underlying concerns. What are your ideas about how these relational barriers can be overcome?*

____

____

____

____

____

____

Profile of Involuntary Psychiatric Patients

Research studies suggest that there is a particular diagnostic and psychosocial functioning profile of involuntary hospital patients. The most whose most common axis I diagnoses' are schizophrenia and bipolar disorder (Hugo, 1999; Hopko et al., 2002; Girolamo et al. 2008; Jarrett et al., 2008; Xiao et al., 2004; Jarrett et al., 2008). Involuntary admits also present with the most severe cognitive impairments, agitation, psychotic symptoms, and propensities for violence (Huber et al., 2012; Hopko et al., 2002; Anestis et al., 2013; Georgieva et al., 2012; Swanson et al., 2003; Hugo, 1999; Zeller, 2010; Xiao et al., 2004; Girolamo et al. 2008; Jarrett et al., 2008).

It is also common to see diagnostic complexity (Xiao et al., 2004). Involuntary admits frequently present with severe substance abuse disorders (Hugo, 1999; Swanson et al., 2003; Watson et al., 2000; Elila et al., 2008; Opsal et al., 2013; Ries et al., 2009). This is of particular concern because substance abuse associates with suicidal ideation and homicidal ideation, which offers a partial explanation for the association between substance abuse and involuntary hospitalization (Opsal et al., 2013; Huber et al., 2012). Co-occurring substance abuse disorders also confound research attempts to study involuntary populations as a homogenous group (Holm et al., 2012). Co-occurring medical conditions are also common amongst involuntary admits and associate with hospital recidivism (Opsal et al., 2013; Lyons et al., 1997).

Involuntary admits present with recurrent psychosocial stressors and impairments in activities of daily living (Hugo, 1999; Girolamo et al., 2008). I have rank ordered these factors according to DSM-V priority in treatment (American Psychological Association, 2013). Involuntary admits frequently are of a low socioeconomic status and education, have employment problems, struggle with psychiatric medication adherence, and often have significant criminal justice histories (Hopko et al., 2002; Swanson et al., 2003; Hugo, 1999; Girolamo et al., 2008; Huber et al., 2012). Severely mentally ill adults who are involuntarily hospitalized are also more likely to be experiencing a first psychotic break or have a more chronic history of hospitalization (Huber et al., 2002; Swanson et al., 2003; Xiao et al., 2004). It is important to add that involuntary admits are often younger, male, living alone, and African American (Xiao et al., 2004; Hopko et al., 2002; Girolamo et al. 2008; Hustoft et al., 2013; Huber et al., 2012; Swanson et al., 2003).

In summary, involuntary adult psychiatric hospital inpatients are frequently men who are the most vulnerable, mentally and substance abuse disordered, impoverished, violent, and psychosocially impaired. This profile is generally consistent with the profile of patients who: commit violence, are hospitalized due to risk of harming others (a relative rarity), feel humiliated in response to being hospitalized, become violent on inpatient units, are involuntarily treated in inpatient settings, abscond from hospitals, and are rehospitalized (Taube, 2013; Hustoft et al., 2013; Tuohimaki et al., 2013; Svindesth et al., 2013; Steinert et al., 2007; Hugo et al., 1999; Winkler et al., 2012; Zeller, 2010; Stellwagen et al., 2010; Jarrett et al., 2008; Lyons et al., 1997; Segal et al., 2008; Zenner et al., 2007). Encouragingly, these findings suggest that patients who are the most at risk are also those who are hospitalized.

Several researchers make recommendations for the treatment of involuntary patients. Rodrigues et al. (2009) notes that they have unique treatment needs and therefore require specialized inpatient units and treatment protocols. Dmitriev et al. (2007) proposes a treatment approach that consists of the following stages: adjustment and diagnosis, intensive treatment and rehabilitation, internalization of therapeutic gains, and discharge. Girolamo et al. (2008) elaborates that involuntary inpatients also require specialized interventions that can help to improve their receptivity, engagement, and adherence to treatment plans.

Positive Outcomes

Frequently, patients resent involuntary care in the short term and regain their capacity in the long term (Anestis et al., 2013). Involuntarily hospitalization may provide highly symptomatic patients with a much needed break from overwhelming life circumstances (Vuckovich et al., 2005; Pesze, 1975). Patients may then change their point of view over time (Hopko et al., 2002). Munetz et al. (2001) describes a shift from a delusional denial of the illness to an increasing level of acceptance that is a “start on a real journey of recovery” (p. 41). Improvements over time include: Increased cooperativeness with treatment, improved GAFF scores, and reduced aggression within 24 hours, no longer seeing involuntary treatment as a negative occurrence within three weeks, decreased perceived coercion in daily interactions within 12 months, and longer term reductions in dangerous behavior (Georgieva et al., 2012; Wallsten et al., 2007; Dianov et al., 2007; Anestis et al., 2013).

With varying levels of gratitude, patients often acknowledge that involuntary treatments restore their safety and humanity (Guarda et al., 2007; Vuckovich et al., 2005; Anestis et al., 2013). As stated by one involuntary patient: "I would have been angry and fought, but if they had stuffed pills down my throat, I would have kissed their asses and thanked them once I got my mind back, because no one wants to be crazy like that" (Earley, 2006, p. 372). Retrospectively, patients often acknowledge that involuntary care was good for them and should be repeated if they decompensate again in the future (Olsen, 2003; Jarrett et al., 2008). Unsurprisingly, positive attitudes about involuntary care are tied to positive outcomes and negative attitudes are tied to negative experiences (Bentley, 2010). Jarret et al. (2008) found that patients who had a positive view of their involuntary treatment experience *and* patients who had a negative view acknowledge that *some people* have emotional problems that they are not aware of and that psychiatric treatment is generally helpful.

Hospitalizing Psychotic Patients

It may be necessary to hospitalize psychotic patients who refuse medications because prompt treatment may prevent irreversible decompensation (Borgeat et al., 2004; Jarrett et al., 2008; Munetz et al., 2001). The latter authors note that this is particularly true for patients with bipolar or schizophrenic disorders. The cognitive symptoms that are characteristic of these disorders may interfere with treatment engagement and adherence. As such, intermittent adherence is common. This is of concern because it may ultimately result in a worsening of their conditions. In such cases, giving patients numerous opportunities to try their own preferred alternatives to medications can ultimately result in a lesser likelihood of a fuller recovery. As stated by Even Hummelvoll, involuntary care for acutely psychotic patients can be considered: "Genuine paternalism" and "a caring deprivation of liberty" (Vuckovich et al., 2005, p.379).

Hospitalizing Eating Disorder Patients

Anorexia is a disorder that compromises self-image and judgment to the point that dangerously underweight patients deprive themselves of food (Guarda et al., 2007). The authors elaborate that this results in high mortality and morbidity rates, which justifies involuntary hospitalization under the medical principle of beneficence.

Frequently, anorexic patients respond positively to forced feeding and other compulsory treatments and then rapidly decompensate after hospital discharge (Holm et al., 2012; Watson et al., 2000; Bryden et al., 2010). Anorexics learn become adept at complying with treatment and tell professionals what they want to hear so as to be released from the hospital and return to their former lifestyles (Guarda et al., 2007; Bryden et al., 2010). Further study is needed to better understand this dilemma from the patient perspective and construct interventions that may ultimately increase voluntary adherence and therefore preserve life.

Hospitalizing Manic Patients

Symptoms of mania include high energy, insomnia, impulsivity, grandiosity, poor insight, and poor judgment (Zeller, 2010). These symptoms often lead to dangerous behavior, neglected self-care, and treatment refusal, which warrants involuntary hospitalization (Spellecy, 2007; Borgeat et al., 2004). The latter authors elaborate that sound-minded patients, family members, and professionals generally agree that manic patients should not have full, independent decision making authority and that involuntary measures may be necessary. The authors acknowledge that patients and interested parties have varying opinions about how decision making authority should be dispersed. This is particularly true when professionals and family members make attempts to hospitalize manic patients, primarily, in order to prevent them from squandering their money (Stewart et al., 2012).

Hospitalizing Substance Abusing Patients

According to official records, substance abusers comprised 27% of emergency psychiatric visits from 1992 – 2000 (Zeller, 2010). They frequently resist and refuse treatment, have the shortest hospital stays, leave hospitals against medical advice, have poor outcomes, and are the most costly subgroup of psychiatric inpatients (Bruns et al., 2009; Ries et al., 2009).

Outcomes are much better when substance abusers are mandated to substance abuse treatment centers (rather than being involuntarily hospitalized). Coercive treatment is often necessary to engage substance abusing patients (Guarda et al., 2007). This is a theme which frequents the stories of recovered Alcoholics faced with losing a job or family (Munetz et al., 2001). It is also a common theme in the treatment of substance abusing mothers and forensic populations (Nace et al., 2007). Positive outcomes of court-mandated treatment include increased: appointment attendance, engagement with treatment resources, self-advocacy in court, and contact with children (Bruns et al., 2012). As in the case of psychiatric patients, mandated substance abusers often retrospectively acknowledge that, in spite of initial resistance, treatment was ultimately good for them (Bourquin-Teiche et al., 2001). Positive outcomes from court-mandated treatment often correlate with positive family factors, including improved family cohesion and communication (McRee et al., 2012; Tolou-Shams et al., 2012).

Negative Outcomes

Involuntary hospitalization can be said to unduly deny patient liberty, privacy, autonomy, dignity, and empowerment (Siponen, 2007; Anestis et al., 2013; Munetz et al., 2001). The latter authors elaborate that involuntary care paternalistically assumes that providers know patients better than patients know themselves. Furthermore, arguments that the positive outcomes of involuntary care justify violations of rights "could be used to justify any number of paternalistic interventions which would and should be considered unjustifiable" (Spellecy, 2007, p. 47).

Hospitalization is also not substantiated to prevent harm (Brophy et al., 2003). It may only delay the occurrence of harm and is certain to decrease the voluntary usage of health services (Xiao et al., 2004). This is particularly true for involuntarily hospitalized schizophrenics who are involuntarily treated with antipsychotics (Hughes et al., 2009; Rodrigues et al., 2009). The disengagement from services is particularly concerning because it predicts poor treatment prognosis and may elevates risk for suicide (Vuckovich et al., 2005; Skeem et al., 2006).

Negative clinical outcomes frequent the literature on involuntary care. Recurring themes include patient demoralization, social stigmatization, and loss of: self-esteem, identity, self-control, self-efficacy, humanity, and recovery (Rymaszewska, 2007; Brophy et al., 2003; Hughes et al., 2009). Involuntary care also associated with less global improvement after discharge, ongoing problems with employment and social functioning, longer term noncompliance, longer durations of hospitalization, and increased likelihood of rehospitalization (Hopko et al., 2002).

Involuntary care also has negative effects on the inpatient treatment process. Patients with histories of coerced treatment are often reluctant to disclose their presenting symptomology to providers, or ask for professional help (Jarrett et al., 2008). The authors elaborate that coerced treatment destroys patient-provider trust and damages therapeutic relationships, particularly when competent patients refuse treatment and are involuntarily medicated. This may offer a partial explanation for why involuntary patients frequently play compliance games (Hughes et al. (2009). This may be a defensive-adaptive reaction to a stressful circumstance such as an unwanted intervention, a maneuver designed to achieve early release, a response to feeling coerced into treatment, or a strategy to avoid seclusions (Wallsten et al., 2007; Olsen, 2003). Negative effects also include decreased ability of sedated patients to participate in treatment or be evaluated for dispositions (Zeller, 2010). Therefore, involuntary care mechanisms can be said to create an environment that elevates risk for various patient abuses and medicalizes human suffering (Brophy et al., 2003). Furthermore, involuntary care may be of more benefit to inpatient staff that are susceptible to finding anti-therapeutic strategies for managing unruly patient behavior (Keller, 2007; Regan, 2010).

Writing Assignment: *Put yourself in the position of a patient who is being involuntarily hospitalized. What do you think this experience might be like? What factors might make it a relatively better experience? What factors might make it a relatively worse experience?*

____

____

____

____

____

____

PATIENT EXPERIENCE OF INVOLUNTARY CARE

Patients often experience hospital environments as unfamiliar and frightening (Andreasson et al., 2012). Treatments that hospital patients receive are often highly intrusive and unwanted (Munetz et al., 2001). As a result, patients often look back on hospitalization as a negative experience (Zeller, 2010). The author notes that negative experiences can have lasting effects on patient desires to seek professional help and adhere to medications. Therefore, it is important to better understand the patient experience of involuntary care so that it can be improved. I will attempt to increase understanding of the patient experience by presenting recurring themes that frequent the scholarly literature. The themes include patient autonomy, relationships with staff, trauamatization, perceived coercion, and humiliation. I will show that increased patient autonomy associates with stronger staff-patient relationships. Decreased autonomy will be shown to predict poorer staff-patient relationships, and more traumatization, perceived coercion, and humiliation.

Autonomy

Maintaining patient autonomy during hospitalization is particularly important because it associates with improvements in psychiatric functioning (Olsen, 2003). Patients feel that their autonomy is maintained when their subjective quality of life is taken seriously by staff, they are made to feel safe, their vulnerabilities are understood, they are helped to understand what is happening to them, they are granted some time away from the ward with non-uniformed staff, they participate in decision-making processes concerning their care, and staff exert no more control over them than is necessary (Swanson et al., 2003; Andreasson et al., 2012). Patient autonomy decreases when they feel more confined and restricted, have fewer opportunities for social interaction, and foresee a bleak recovery process (Hughes et al., 2009).

It is particularly important for patient autonomy to be respected as much as possible during the process of administering involuntary medications. When involuntarily medicated, patients feel panic, anger, sadness, powerlessness, relief, fear, and develop a particular fear of refusing medications in the future (Jarrett et al., 2008). Giving patients the choice of a less intrusive method of taking medication can help to mediate the negative experience and lessen the likelihood of a violent response (Vuckovich et al., 2005).

Relationships with Staff

Patient-staff relationships are important because they indirectly predict treatment outcomes (Hughes et al., 2009). The authors elaborate that patients maintain their sense of self through relationships with providers. The authors also note that patient loss of sense of self is a major barrier to recovery. The presence of working alliances often depends on the level of staff education, awareness, and training (Rydelius, 2007). Contrastingly, patient-staff conflicts often result in patient attempts to abscond (Zenner et al., 2007).

Zeller (2010) describes positive staff-patient relationships as developing as a result of compassionate and collaborative efforts to engage patients who are in states of crisis. The author adds that the early establishment of working alliances has been found to predict better outcomes and decrease the likelihood of violent behavior on inpatient units. In order for working alliances to develop, patients must experience staff as reliable, attentive, committed, concerned, experienced, humorous, competent, non-rejecting in response to help seeking behavior, emotionally close to patients yet respectful of their needs for solitude, and oriented to firmness, fairness, and stability (Andreasson et al., 2012).

Andreasson et al. (2012) elaborate that staff-patient working alliances promote trust and hope in the treatment process. Alliances also help patients assimilate treatment-related information. Patients need information that reflects reality, including tactful deliverance of information about their illnesses and treatment options, as well as possible consequences of refusing medication. Such transparent dialogue helps patients develop new insights, reduces patient anxieties, and defuses potentially threatening situations. Similarly, Berry et al. (2002) confirms an association between the manner in which health-related information is delivered to patients and patient adherence to treatment plans.

Patient Satisfaction

Mental health services are increasingly being evaluated according to levels of patient satisfaction (Ruggeri, 1994; Swanson et al., 2003). Satisfaction has been found to predict treatment adherence, outcome, and hospital recidivism (Boyer et al., 2009; Druss et al., 1999). Satisfaction also associates with patient autonomy and relationships with staff (Ruggeri, 1994; Boydell et al., 2010; Hughes et al., 2009). These associations provide a strong base of research for my study. Encouragingly, research supports that the majority of involuntary inpatients are satisfied with their care (Hughes et al., 2009). The authors elaborate that patients frequently report high levels of satisfaction in retrospect after they discharge.

In order to feel more satisfied with treatment, patients need to experience the hospital environment as warm, friendly, adequate, safe, comfortable, and based on reasonable rules (Rydelius, 2007; Andreasson et al., 2012). The latter authors elaborate that patients need help settling into daily routines and getting involved in daily activities. Less verbal patients can be engaged through nonverbal activities such as making art projects, taking walks, and playing games. Patients particularly appreciate opportunities to leave the ward, which helps them prepare for a more structured life once they discharge. Sources of patient dissatisfaction include the disruptions caused by threatening and violent patients, receiving treatment with patients from different diagnostic categories, being moved to different units, and lacking structured activities.

Traumatization

The stripping of involuntary patient autonomy, privacy, and self-esteem can be traumatizing for both for patients and staff (Andreasson et al., 2012; Huber et al., 2012; Georgieva et al., 2012). In particular, patients report that being strapped down and having their clothes taken off so as to be involuntarily medicated makes them feel as if they are being raped (Hughes et al., 2009). Involuntary mechanisms are often implemented so as to prevent violence, though paradoxically provoke violent responses (Lebel, 2007).

Negative effects have lead government officials to advocate for the reduction or even elimination of involuntary treatments (Stellwagen et al., 2010). Traumatization can be prevented by reduced usage of seclusion, restraint, and increased patient participation in treatment (Regan, 2010). It can also be reduced by orienting hospital treatment to patients' strengths and debriefing with patients after involuntary treatments are administered (Andreasson et al., 2012).

Perceived Coercion

Studies of perceived coercion help to illuminate the difference between the reality of particular inpatient hospital situations and how those situations are perceived by patients, which can strongly influence patient behavior and corresponding treatment outcomes (Andreasson et al., 2012). Patients who perceive less coercion tend to feel respected, treated fairly, and more involved in decision making processes concerning their treatment (Anestis et al., 2013). Munetz et al. (2001) calls this *procedural justice*. Patients who perceive more coercion generally feel that treatment decisions are made for them and do not meaningfully consider their perspectives (Guarda et al., 2007; Svindseth et al., 2013). Higher levels of perceived coercion associates with a) poorer therapeutic alliances b) poorer therapeutic outcomes c) increased vulnerability to traumatizing effects and d) variable effects on engagement with psychiatric services (Zeller, 210; Swanson et al., 2003; Anestis et al., 2013; Georgieva et al., 2012; Guarda et al., 2007).

Studies of perceived coercion are also important from a legal-ethical perspective because hospital patients are in a vulnerable position and thereby susceptible to manipulation at the hands of professional power (Reamer et al., 1990). High levels of perceived coercion associate with the negative effects of institutionalization on personality, the patient's previous inpatient hospital experiences, staff putting psychological pressure on patients prior to the administration of involuntary treatment, and a hostile-dominant interpersonal style that often develops in response (Anestis et al., 2013; Georgieva et al., 2012). The latter authors elaborate that staff pressure may exacerbate patients' pre-existing paranoia or psychotic symptoms that are targeted for decrease. Similarly, Mendel et al. (2011) found that more directive physician approaches can lead impressionable patients to disregard what they know works for them. This may ultimately result in poorer satisfaction and lower levels of adherence.

Vulnerable population factors also appear in the perceived coercion literature. Anestis et al. (2013) found that women perceived significantly more coercion than men. This may relate to women's (generally greater) emotional responsiveness (Georgieva et al., 2012). Adhering to medications has been found to help adults with schizophrenia cope with high levels of perceived coercion (Bentley, 2010).

Humiliation

Humiliation can be thought of as the emotional expression of perceived coercion and is reported by patients to associate with involuntary confinement in and of itself (Svindseth et al., 2013). It also associates with the patient perception of staff abuses of power and the traumatizing process of being involuntarily medicated described previously (Andreasson et al., 2012; Vuckovich et al., 2005).

The factors that were noted to increase patient autonomy generally reduce humiliation. This includes presenting patients with options for treatment, increasing their opportunities to make choices, helping patients accept treatment options rather than utilizing coercive tactics, giving patients ample time to introspect about their presenting circumstances, and having caring discussions with staff (Andreasson et al., 2012). Such discussions can be particularly helpful to patients who report feeling humiliated during the admission process (Svindseth et al., 2013).

Vulnerable Populations

Cultural values may strongly influence patient acknowledgement of mental illness and willingness to seek treatment (Townsend, 2009). Studies confirm that rates of severe mental illness are especially high among ethnic minorities (Schnittker, 2003). They have less access to mental health services, receive poorer quality services, carry a greater burden as a result of their psychiatric conditions, and consequentially utilize high numbers of emergency mental health services (Eack et al., 2012; Camacho et al., 2012). These factors associate with a lower quality of life and increase risk for psychiatric hospitalization (Swanson et al., 2003; Camacho et al., 2012). This discussion offers support for Eack et al.'s (2012) position that further study is needed on minority help-seeking and protective factors. The author notes that these factors help to reduce risk and increase service linkages.

African Americans

"Research has consistently documented black-white differences in rates of voluntary psychiatric treatment that cannot be reduced entirely to differences in either access or need," (Schnittker, 2003, p. 506). The author notes that African Americans have comparable rates of mental illness compared to Caucasians, yet only 16% of African Americans who need mental health treatment actually receive it. The author adds that most services they do receive are inappropriate for their needs. Eack et al. (2012) adds that, after adjusting for socioeconomic and other demographic variables, African Americans tend to discharge from inpatient psychiatric hospitals with lower symptom improvements and are less likely to become employed.

This offers a plausible explanation for why African Americans' are generally less satisfied with inpatient treatments and psychiatric medications in particular (Boydell et al., 2010; Schnittker, 2003). This may also offer an explanation for why African Americans are generally reluctant to seek mental health services, as stated by the latter authors.

Consequentially, African Americans are also more likely to utilize emergency services and be involuntarily hospitalized (Catalano et al., 2007; Tolmac et al., 2004; Camacho et al., 2012; Eack et al., 2012).

African Americans frequently receive a different standard of care from other cultural minorities (Schnittker, 2003). The author notes that this partially relates to African American communities lacking resources to put toward mental health services, lacking health insurance, and relying on inadequate public programs. African Americans also disproportionately receive injectable, antipsychotic, and involuntary medications (Eack et al., 2012; Jarrett et al., 2008). The latter authors thoroughly adjusted odds ratios based on reasons for detention, risk of violence, assault on staff, absconding attempts, drug and alcohol use, and agitation. The authors concluded that it was unlikely that providers were providing discriminatory treatment based on stereotypes.

There are several plausible explanations for the aforementioned disparities that may be at least partially true. Camacho et al. (2012) explains these disparities as relating to African Americans' reluctance to seek treatment until symptoms are sufficiently severe, nonadherence with treatment plans, and high drop-out rates. Schnittker (2003) contests such arguments on the basis that "whites have historically been the disproportionate beneficiaries of medical improvements" and are therefore more broadly enthusiastic (p. 518).

Camacho et al. (2012) noted that African Americans are frequently misdiagnosed with psychotic disorders. Eack et al. (2012) elaborates that these misdiagnoses' often form the basis of detention, though there is little to no difference in actual prevalence rates of psychotic disorders in African American and non-African American populations. Catalano et al. (2007) noted that African Americans are particularly impacted by rising unemployment rates. These rising rates associate with increased hospitalizations for nonviolent, public nuisance behavior that arguably meets criteria for civil commitment.

Schnittker (2003) clarifies that African Americans do not generally dismiss medical models of illness and treatment in their entirety. They also do not rely more heavily on spiritual explanations of mental illness. Rather, they hesitate to endorse narrow explanations of mental illness as being caused exclusively by family dysfunction or genetic factors. The authors elaborate that these latter explanations may be reminiscent of racist ideologies and historically maleficent treatments.

Psychiatric Medications

A prominent factor in patient vulnerability is medication adherence. The process of giving and taking medication may seem simple, though it is a complicated and richly dynamic process (Bentley, 2010). According to a drug-centered model, drugs are psychoactive and therefore alter physical and mental states, a consequence that amounts to the therapeutic effects of the prescription (Allison, 2012). People use drugs to fix a multitude of social, psychological, financial, and emotional problems on the premise that those problems have neurological underpinnings (Cohen, 2008).

Drug effects are influenced by patient experiences, history, norms, status, roles, faith and hope, peer opinions, and various influences by advertising (Cohen, 2008). The author elaborates that the relative goodness or badness of a drug effect may be a point of view, such as when a patient takes benzodiazepines and then experiences relief from anxiety *or* sedation. This is important because patient interpretations of drug effects have a strong influence on adherence and outcomes (Bentley, 2010). The author elaborates that this is why practitioners and researchers need to know about the lived experience of consumers taking medications, which consumers often have deep desires to be heard about.

Psychiatric medications profoundly influence patients' sense of self, identity, and life experiences (Roe et al., 2009; Cohen, 2008; Bentley, 2010). The latter author notes that patients who take psychiatric medications must internally and externally negotiate issues of resistance, acceptance, and dependence. Medication can be "an avenue to full humanness and a more positive life experience, but can also be the source of felt differentness and resignation," (p. 488).

Writing Assignment: *What are your beliefs, in general, about psychiatric medications? If you were meeting with an adult male with schizophrenia for individual therapy who refused to take medications in spite of chronic, involuntary hospitalizations, how might your core beliefs about medication benefit his treatment? How might your beliefs be a liability to his treatment?*

____

____

____

____

____

____

Now that I have presented a basic overview of medication effects, I will present some history on the subject. In the 1960's and 70's, medications were psychodynamically formulated as a symbol of nurturance and power in the patient-psychiatrist dyad (Bentley, 2010). By the 1980's, psychiatry had established its leadership in mental health (Cohen, 2008). The author elaborates that on the prevailing opinion that distress, dysfunction, and behavioral problems were mere symptoms of biological abnormalities. Accordingly, there was an increase in public and private funding for neurobiology and drug treatments. The author noted that, by the year 2000, 13% of middle aged women in America were taking anti-depressants. Over the last decade, the use of medications has grown drastically (Covell et al., 2007). Prescribing two or more medications is now the standard rather than a rarity (Townsend, 2009).

In spite of increasing usage, medications have resulted in widespread negative outcomes that are discussed by Cohen (2008). Several studies report that antidepressants sometimes result in longer and more frequent depressive episodes. Longitudinal research findings indicate that the symptom remission rates for schizophrenia in 1992 were no better than in the 1920's when hydrotherapy predominated. The number of individuals in the United States who received social security benefits for mental disorders increased from 3.505 million in 1987 to 5.77 million in 2002, a64% increase. According to data published by the World Bank (2013), this is nearly four times the 16.1% total population growth of that time period. This could mean that the relative number of severely mentally ill individuals is growing faster than the population, though it could also mean that the system is doing a better job of identifying mentally ill individuals and providing them with resources. Cohen (2008) disclaimers that negative findings on medications do not suggest that they sustain or exacerbate dysfunction, though aggregate data suggests that medications fail to decrease dysfunction *on the whole*. Research on medications that claims positive outcomes should also be scrutinized in light of pharmaceutical companies tainting clinical trials and publications.

With varying levels of reliability, research generally supports that medications decrease psychiatric symptoms (Roe et al., 2009). Medication does not cure symptoms, but does provide some relief (Allison, 2012). Psychiatric medications frequently have positive neurological effects, improve cognitions, and positively affect psychological and emotional functioning (Bentley, 2010). The author notes that medications may also help patients achieve goals, maintain identify, and avoid unwanted outcomes such as hospitalization.

Provider Approaches to Medication Management

When we prioritize drugs over other forms of help, we label economic, emotional, spiritual, psychological, and educational problems as diseases (Cohen, 2008). The author notes that this phenomenon is commonly known as medicalization (Cohen, 2008). A medical model of psychiatry unjustifiably imposes assumptions about the capacity of mentally ill patients (Allison, 2012).The author elaborates that a traditional medical model decreases patient willingness to talk to providers about what they find helpful. Consequentially, the medical model approach is not satisfying to many patients. Nevertheless, the approach continues to guide contemporary psychiatric practice. This is at least partially due to the influence of the pharmaceutical industry on policy and training.

The medical model of psychiatry traditionally views patients' responses to interventions as either compliant or noncompliant. This is largely based on physician theories about proper patient behavior, medical professional authority, and hierarchical patient-physician relationships (Roe et al., 2009). Under the medical model of care, patients are often pressured to take medications that they may have reservations about (Allison, 2012). Deegan (2007) considers this paternalistic, subjugating, disrespectful, and unrealistic. As she notes on p. 63, "framing complex human behavior in simplistic terms of compliance versus noncompliance often obscures more than it reveals."

Patients making choices concerning their treatment is central to *shared decision making*, an alternative to traditional compliance models (Deegan, 2007). Shared decision making may help to decrease the negative effects associated with patient expectations about medications (Roe et al., 2009; Faase et al., 2012). Encouragingly, providers are generally becoming more transparent in medication management sessions (Bentley, 2010). The author also notes that providers are generally decreasing the hierarchical nature of patient-provider relationships in order to hear the patient voice. This discussion underscores researcher advocacy for a more egalitarian view of medications and therapeutic dialogue (Cohen, 2008; Hughes et al., 2009).

Patients need an open, safe, and supportive forum to discuss their concerns about medications without pressure from professionals (Roe et al., 2009). Patient perspectives on medications should be elicited through collaborative approaches discussed by Townsend

(2009). First, stigma must be overcome and patients must develop a fundamental understanding of their illness, relapse triggers, and the role of medication adherence in their recoveries. Motivational interviewing can help to explore stigma and social environment influences on adherence. This can help to set the stage for CBT interventions that attempt to increase adherence.

Educating patients about treatment options and efficacy is part of responsible, evidence-based practice (Townsend, 2009). Patients need evidence-based information about medications in order to accurately weigh risks and benefits (Dyck et al., 2005). This includes the exploration of risks associated with taking medications as well as the risks associated with not taking medications (Zikmund-Fischer, 2008). The author elaborates that risks should be explained to patients in realistic terms, which helps to decrease irrational worries. For example, explaining that a particular medication *increases risk by 50%* exaggerates an elevation in risk from 2% to 3%. Dyck et al. (2005) cautions that providing patients with *too much* information can also result in overload, anxiety, and frustration.

Medications have only a limited contribution to the longer term prognosis for mental health recovery (Allison, 2012).Mental health consumers and related stake holders are increasingly insisting on interventions that are more acceptable and worthwhile to them (Swanson et al., 2003). The authors elaborate that psychiatric treatments are unlikely to be adhered to if they merely control symptoms and do not lead to a more meaningful recovery.

Deegan (2007) discusses *personal medicine*, which are activities that are meaningful to patients and therefore essential to their recoveries. Personal medicine may consistent of learning and developing unique talents, employment, and engaging in intimate relationships. For example, a patient tells his psychiatrist: "My marriage is powerful personal medicine, and is the most important thing in my life. I don't want paranoia or sexual side effects to stress my marriage. You and I have to find a medication that supports me in my marriage so my marriage can support my recovery," (p. 65). The author elaborates on recovery principles of care, including that goals of medication adherence should be recovery and not maintenance, psychiatric medicine should serve personal medicine, and that the treatment team should support patients through their difficulties in order to achieve optimal benefits of traditional medicine and personal medicine.

Medication Adherence

Whether or not patients take psychiatric medications as prescribed is contemporarily regarded as *adherence*, a more patient-centered alternative to traditional notions of compliance (Roe et al., 2009). Full adherence to medications as prescribed is necessary to receive the maximum benefit possible and reduce risk of hospitalization (DiBonaventura et al., 2012).

Rates of medication adherence among the severely mentally ill are generally 30 – 50% (Allison, 2012; Roe, 2009; Deegan, 2007). Research supports a link between non-adherence and: poor insight into illness, increased medication side effects, substance use and abuse, violence, high risk behavior, lower quality of life, family members bearing a more significant economic burden, a chaotic life style, symptom relapse and chronicity, and increased rates of completed suicide (Townsend, 2009; Jarrett et al., 2008; Roe et al., 2009). Nonadherence is often followed by hospitalization, and substantially increases health care service usage and related costs (Camacho et al., 2012; Swanson et al., 2003; DiBonaventura et al., 2012).

It is important to understand patient attitudes, cultural values, contextual cues, feelings, and subjective experiences that influence decisions about whether or not to adhere to medication regiments (Roe et al., 2009; Covell et al., 2007). Patients may stop taking medications for fear that others will find out, employment or personal relationships will be jeopardized, lack of funds to pay for medications, fear of health complications, a desire for culturally-based or spiritual solutions, viewing medication usage as a sign of weakness, lacking a reason to get well, medications may be unwanted reminders of having an illness, not considering ones' self mentally ill enough to require medications, and medications may negatively impact quality of life in a more general way (Deegan, 2007; Jarrett et al., 2008). Patients with transportation problems may also have difficulty attending appointments and obtaining prescriptions from pharmacies (Townsend, 2009). Nearly half of patients in a research study reported that they sometimes forget to take their medication (DiBonaventura et al., 2012). The authors found that non-adherent patients were less likely to be married, employed, or college educated. Roe et al. (2009) reports that non-adherence more often reflects a disagreement between patient and provider, rather than poor judgment on the part of the patient.

Roe et al. (2009) conceptualize the decision to stop taking medications as occurring in a five stage process. The stages include a) the occurrence of a major emotional crisis b) negative consequences and experiences with medications are more particularly noticed, including the loss of personality c) there is conflict between personal desire to stop taking medications and pressure from supportive others to continue taking medications d) the conflict and underlying ambivalence is gradually resolved (sometimes in secret), and e) a personal perspective on taking medications is developed. This may result in a decision to stop medications, though patients who discontinue may be open to taking medications in the future as needed.

Antipsychotics

Antipsychotics continue to be a cornerstone of treatment for serious psychiatric conditions (Meehan et al., 2011). The authors note that they help psychotic patients stabilize and reduce risk of symptom relapse. Antipsychotic treatments for schizophrenia frequently improve patient quality of life and productivity (DiBonaventura et al., 2012).

In spite of the benefits of adherence, rates of patient discontinuation of antipsychotics are high (Covell et al., 2007). Adherence rates for adults with schizophrenia may be even lower than the 30-50% rate quoted previously (Garcia et al., 2006; Townsend, 2009). Total costs of hospitalization associated with non-adherence to antipsychotic medication are estimated at between $1.4 and $1.8 billion (DiBonaventura et al., 2012). Morrison et al. (2000) found that nonadherence with antipsychotics was a critical factor in 92% of patient hospital readmissions.

Nonadherence with antipsychotics often relates to the severity of side effects (DiBonaventura et al., 2012). The side effects of older antipsychotics profoundly lowered patient quality of life, sometimes causing even greater distress than the illnesses themselves (Morrison et al., 2000). Patients taking older antipsychotics often report that they feel strange, sedated, and lose their will power, coherent thinking, and spontaneity (Covell et al., 2007). Akathisia, or inner restlessness, is a particularly powerful side effect of older antipsychotics (Jarrett et al., 2008).

Patients overwhelmingly prefer the recently invented atypical antipsychotics due to less severe side effects (Townsend, 2009; Covell et al., 2007). The latter authors elaborate that atypical antipsychotics are less likely to result in parkinsonian symptoms, tardive dyskinesia, and akathisia. However, newer antipsychotics may cause weight gain, increased risk of diabetes, hyperlipidemia, and sexual dysfunction. Other side effects such as tremors, stiffness, drooling, restlessness and shaking can affect patient motor, psychological, and social functioning (Meehan et al., 2011). The authors note that side effects of antipsychotics may also exacerbate pre-existing symptomology and risk for mental health relapse.

Meehan et al., (2011) conducted a study of adults with schizophrenia taking antipsychotics and found that there were almost equal numbers of patients who experienced no side effects and patients who experienced severe side effects. Most patients under study did not report sexual side effects, though males comprised 73% of the sample and therefore may not have reported accurately due to embarrassment.

Side Effects

Patients have complained about medication side effects throughout history, though these complaints have only begun to be taken seriously in recent history (Morrison et al., 2000). 80-90% of the severely mentally ill report at least one bothersome side effect (DiBonaventura et al., 2012; Covell et al., 2007). The latter authors note that addressing patient experiences of side effects may result in improved medication treatments plans, adherence, patient-provider communication, and outcomes. The patient experience of side effects may vary depending on the number and severity of side effects, as well as patient expectations of medication effects, severity of illness, and anxiety (Berry et al., 2002; Covell et al., 2007; Faase et al., 2012).

Morrison et al. (2000) describes side effects as unpleasant, emotionally draining, and causing of distress. In particular, involuntary patients (who frequently receive more intrusive medications) describe side effects as frightening and powerful (Hughes et al., 2009). Research supports that patients are most concerned about medication effects on their sleep, as well as restlessness, trouble concentrating, sedation, dry mouth, drooling, dizziness, and weight gain (Bentley, 2010; DiBonaventura et al., 2012; Meehan et al., 2011; Covell et al., 2007). The latter authors report that weight gain is a particular concern for non-African American women. This is consistent with research findings that confirm less that African Americans are generally less concerned about thinness. The latter authors also note that men are most significantly concerned about sexual side effects.

The severity of side effects has been found to predict lower medication adherence in multiple studies (Deegan, 2007; Allison, 2012; Townsend, 2009; Faase, et al., 2012). In one study, the number of patients who discontinued medications due to side effects was about twice as high as the number of patients who discontinued due to lack of treatment response (Covell et al., 2007). The side effects that are the most predictive of non-adherence include weight gain, cognitive impairment, agitation, sedation, and metabolic effects (DiBonaventura et al., 2012). Patients are generally less adherent to medications that interfere with personal goals such as working, exercising, and keeping busy (Roe et al., 2009). Therefore, patients who choose not to take medications because of side effects are making a somewhat rationale decision (Morrison et al., 2000). Other factors that predict nonadherence include mistaking illness symptoms for side effects and over-focus on side effects (Meehan et al., 2011; Andreasson et al., 2012).

How providers communicate information to patients about side effects strongly influences adherence (Berry et al., 2002). The authors elaborate that patients tend to calculate the risk of a particular drug according to number of side effects, severity, and likelihood of occurrence. Risks of experiencing side effects should therefore be communicated in percentages when possible, which helps to reduce patient overestimation of vague descriptors such as *rare* or *sometimes* (Dyck et al., 2005). The authors recommend giving patients written pamphlet information on medications that includes information on side effects.

Writing Assignment: *Consider what you have read about the pros, cons, and patient experience of medications and side effects. Put yourself in the position of a patient with a chronic, debilitating psychiatric illness. The patients' symptoms fully remit when medications are taken as prescribed, though the patient feels chronically fatigued, internally restless, emotionally deadened, drools, and shakes. These side effects are prominent enough to attract the attention of others. When the patient does not take medications, the patient is involuntarily hospitalized frequently, cannot work, and is completely isolated from relationships. If you were this patient and were faced with this decision, what would you probably decide and why?*

Coping with Side Effects

Combining side effect management strategies with traditional medical approaches is consistent with a recovery and holistic model of practice (Meehan et al., 2011). Patient ability to manage side effects is also predictive of medication adherence (Berry et al., 2002).

Learning skills to cope with symptoms is essential for mental health recovery (Deegan, 2007). The author emphasizes skills such as using headphones and ear plugs to manage voices, exercising, and meditating. The author note that patients who learn to use one skill are often empowered to learn and use additional skills. Skills include attending gym to combat weight gain, being referred to a dietician, deep breathing and relaxation, referral to a psychologist to develop positive self-talk, diet change to reduce constipation, using powder for itchy skin, watching TV as a distraction, gardening, taking brief rest periods during the day, obtaining prescriptions for valium or cogentin, and obtaining doctor assessment of tongue movement (Morrison et al., 2000).

Meehan et al. (2011) describes a multitude of consumer-recommended strategies. To manage sedation and tiredness, consumers recommend establishing a normal day and night routine, taking short naps in the morning, finding a personally meaningful reason to get up in the morning, splashing water on the face to awaken, having coffee and/or an apple in the morning, taking evening medication 30 minutes prior to bedtime, and thinking positively. Consumers caution against staying in bed late into the morning, napping during the day or evening, watching TV in bed, exercising or eating large meals prior to bedtime, or drinking coffee or tea late in the afternoon or evening. To manage weight gain, consumers recommend eating smaller meals throughout the day, carrying an apply or other piece of fruit to manage snacking urges, sucking on ice cubes made from juice, incorporating exercise into daily routines, avoiding boredom, cooking ones' own food, substituting low fat and low sugar food for high fat and high sugar foods, avoiding keeping chocolate in the home, and not giving in to weight gain.

LIMITATIONS OF EXISTING RESEARCH

Research on involuntary care is often limited by differences between participants and nonparticipants, the impossibility of random assignment, design flaws, and data reporting problems. Nonparticipants are generally more seriously mentally ill, diagnosed with schizophrenia, and are less compliant and less satisfied with treatment (Georgieva et al., 2012; Guarda et al., 2007; Boydell et al., 2010). Highly sophisticated treatment-control designs are not possible due to the legality of involuntary care and the ethics of treating patients with histories of violence (Georgieva et al., 2012; Swanson et al., 2003). Studies often have small sample sizes (Hughes et al., 2009; Steinert, 2007; Georgieva et al., 2012; Camacho et al., 2012). Studies are also limited by inaccuracy in patient self-report as well as exclusive reliance on patient self-report or official reports (Hopko et al., 2002; Holm et al., 2012; Tuohimaki et al., 2003; Watson et al., 2000; Lindellus, 2012; Bindman et al., 2002; Tolou-Shams et al., 2012; Bruns et al., 2012). These limitations may offer a partial explanation for the limited generalizeability of research findings on the subject (Camacho et al., 2012). However, ". . . this does not excuse researchers in this field from increasing their efforts to find such data" (Salize et al., 2011, p. 119).

REFERENCES

Adkins, A. (2010). *Help-seeking patterns of African-Americans: Variables that affect professional help seeking* (Doctoral dissertation).

African American Therapists. (2008, December 14). Re: African Americans and Therapy [Online posting] Retrieved from: http://www.africanamericantherapists.com/ Therapy%20&%20Race.htm

Ainsworth, M., Blehar, M., Waters, E., & Wall, S. (1978). *Patterns of attachment: A psychological study of the strange situation.* Hillsdale, NJ: Lawrence Erlbaum Associates Inc.

Ahktar, S. (1995). *A primer of understanding of treating severe personality disorders.* Northvale, NJ: Jason Aronson Publishers Inc.

Alleyne, A. (2004). Black identity and workplace oppression. *Counseling and Psychotherapy Research, 1*(4), 4-8.

Alleyne, A. (2004). The internal oppressor and black identity wounding. *Counseling and Psychotherapy Research, 10*(15), 31-88.

Alim, T., Graves, E., Mellman, T., Aigbogun, E., Gray, E., Lawson, W., & Charney, D. (2006). Trauma exposure, posttraumatic stress disorder, and depression in an African-American primary care setting. *Journal of Medical Association, 8*(10), 1630-1636.

Allison, R., (2012). Promoting a discussion about adherence to psychiatric medication. *Mental Health Practice, 16*(3), 18 -22.

American Psychological Association. (2000). *Diagnostic and statistical manual of mental disorders* (4th ed.). Washington D.C. First, M., Frances, A., Pincus, H., & Widiger, T.

American Psychological Association. (2013). *Diagnostic and statistical manual of mental disorders (5th Ed). Washington*, DC.

American Psychological Association. (2013). Riese f. St. Mary's Hospital and Medical Center, 751 P.2nd 893. Retrieved from: www.apa.or/about/offices/og c/ amicus/riese.aspx The American Psychologist. (2005, November). *Enhancing professional competence through developmental approaches to supervision.* Washington, D.C.: Stoltenberg, C.

Andreasson, E., & Skarsater, I. (2012). Patients' treated for psychosis and their perceptions of care in compulsory treatment: Basis for an action plan. *Journal of Psychiatric and Mental Health Nursing, 19,* 15 – 22.

Anestis, A. (2013). Predictors of perceived coercion in patients admitted for psychiatric hospitalization and the stability of these perceptions over time. *Psychiatry, Psychology, and the Law, 20*(4), 492 – 503.

Applegate, J., & Shapiro, J. (2005). *Neurobiology for clinical social work: Theory and practice.* New York, NY: W.W. Norton & Company.

Baecht, L. (2009). Federal courts' interpretations of Sell v. U.S. *The Journal of Psychiatry & Law, 37*, 413 – 30.

Baptiste, D. (2005). Family therapy with East Indian immigrant parents rearing children in the United States: Parental concerns, therapeutic issues, and recommendations. *Contemporary Family Therapy, 27*(3), 345 – 366.

Bateman, A., & Fonagy, P. (2003). The development of an attachment-based treatment program for borderline personality disorder. *Bulletin of the Menninger Clinic. 67*(3), 187 – 211.

Beach, S., Brody, G., Lei, M., & Philibert, R. (2010). Differential susceptibility to parenting among African American youths: Testing the *DRD4* hypothesis. *Journal of Family Psychology, 24*(5), 513 – 521.

Beaulaurier, R (2001). Legislators' view regarding the privatization of involuntary treatment: Implications for mental health administrators. *Administration in Social Work, 25*(4), 47 – 60.

Beck, A. (1973). *Cognitive therapy and the emotional disorders.* New York, NY: The International Universities Press.

Beck, A., Freeman, A., Davis, D., & Associates (2004). *Cognitive therapy of personality Disorder* (2nd ed.). New York, NY: The Guliford Press.

Becker, S., & Curry, J. (2008). Outpatient interventions for adolescent substance abuse: A quality of evidence review. *Journal of Consulting and Clinical Psychology, 76*(4), 531 – 543.

Bellak, L., Hurvich, M., & Gediman, H. (1989). The broad role of ego functions assessment. *The American Journal of Psychiatry, 133*(11), 1259-1264.

Bellak, L., Hurvich, M., & Gediman, H. (1973). *Ego functions in schizophrenics, neurotics, and normals.* Hoboken, NJ: John Wiley & Sons, Inc.

Bellow, G. (2009, December). *Attachment theory and child protective practice.* Paper presented at The Sanville Convocation, Los Angeles, CA.

Benard, B. (2004). *Resiliency: What have we learned.* San Francisco, CA: WestEd Publishing Inc.

Bennett, S. (2006). Clinical writing of a therapy in progress: Ethical questions and therapeutic challenges. *Clinical Social Work Journal, 34*(2), 215-226.

Bentley, K. (2010). Psychiatric medication and meaning-making in a residential program for adults with serious mental illness. *Qualitative Social Work, 9*(4), 479 - 99.

Bernsetin, P. (1988). Patients' rights manual for mental health service providers. *California Association of Mental Health Patient's rights Advocates Training Program.*

Berry, D., Michas, I., & Bersellini, E. (2002). Communicating information about medication side effects: Effects on satisfaction, perceived risk to health, and intent to comply. *Psychology and Health, 17*(3), 247 – 67.

Bindman, J., Tighe, J., Thornicroft, G., & Leese, M. (2002). Poverty, poor service, and compulsory psychiatric treatment in England. *Social Psychiatric Epidemiology, 37,* 341 – 45.

Bjorklund, P. (2000). Assessing ego functioning: Spinning straw into gold. *Perspectives in Psychiatric Care, 36*(1), 14-24.

Blanck, G., & Blanck, R. (1994). *Ego Psychology: Theory and practice* (2nd ed.). New York,

NY: The New York Press.

Blaustein, M., & Kinniburgh, K. (2005). Providing the family as a secure base for therapy with children and adolescents. *Attachment Theory into Practice, 10*(1), 48-53.

Borgeat, F., & Zullino, D. (2004). Attitudes concerning involuntary treatment of mania: Results of a survey within self-help organizations. *European Psychiatry, 19,* 155 – 158.

Bourquin-Tieche, D., Besson, J., Lambert, H., & Yersin, B. (2001). Involuntary treatment of alcohol-dependent patients: A Study of 17 consecutive cases of civil commitment. *Journal of European Addiction Research, 7,* 48 – 55.

Bowlby, J. (1960). Grief and mourning in early infancy and childhood. *The Psychoanalytic Study of the Child, 15,* 9-52.

Bowlby, J. (1963). *Child care and the growth of love.* Baltimore, MA: Penguin Books.

Bowlby, J. (1969). *Attachment and* loss: *Volume* 1. Lubbock, TX: The Hogarth Press & The Institute of Psychoanalysis.

Boydell, J., Morgan, C., Dutta, R., Jones, B., Alemseged, F., Dazzan, P., Morgan, K., Doody, G., Harrison, G., Leff, J., Jones, P., Murray, R., & Fearon, P. (2010). Satisfaction with inpatient treatment for first-episode psychosis among different ethnic groups: A Report from the UK/ESOP study. *International Journal of Social Psychiatry, 58*(1), 98 – 105.

Boyer, L., Baumstarck-Barrau, K., Cano, N., Zendjidjian, X., Belzeaux, R., Limousin, S., Magalon, D., Samuelian, J., Lancon, C., & Auquier, P. (2009). Assessment of psychiatric inpatient satisfaction: A systematic review of self-reported instruments. *European Psychiatry, 24*(8), 540 – 9.

Boyle, S., Hull, G., Mather, J., Smith, L., & Farley, O. (2006). *Direct practice in social work.* Upper Saddle River, NJ: Pearson Education.

Breneman, D. (2004). Forcible antipsychotic medication and the unfortunate side effects of Sell v. United States. *Harvard Journal of Law and Public Policy, 27,* 965 – 84.

Bridges, N. (2006). Clinical writing about patients: Negotiating the impact on patients and their treatment. *Journal of Psychoanalytic Social Work, 14*(1), 23-41.

Briere, J., & Spinazzola, J. (2005). Phenomenology and psychological assessment of complex posttraumatic stress. *Journal of Traumatic Stress, 18*(5), 401-412.

Brophy, L., & McDermott, F. (2003). What's driving involuntary treatment in the community? The social, policy, legal, and ethical context. *Australian Psychiatry, 111,* 84 – 90.

Bruns, E., Pullmann, M., Weathers, E., Wirschem, M., & Murphy, J. (2012). Effects of multidimensional family treatment drug court on child and family outcomes: Results of a quasi-experimental study. *Journal of Child Maltreatment, 17*(3), 218 – 230.

Bryden, P., Steinegger, C., & Jarvis, D. (2010). The Ontario experience of involuntary treatment of pediatric patients with eating disorders. *International Journal of Law and Psychiatry, 33,* 138 – 143.

Burstein, M., Stanger, C., Kamon, J., & Dumenci, L. (2006). Parent psychopathology, parenting, and child internalizing problems in substance-abusing families. *Psychology of Addictive Behaviors, 20*(2), 97 – 106.

Butts, H. (2002). The black mask of humanity: Racial/ethnic discrimination and posttraumatic stress disorder. *The Journal of the American Academy of Psychiatry and Law, 30*(3) 336-339.

California Department of Alcohol and Drug Programs. (2010). Grant, G. (2010). *Using trauma informed AOD treatment practices to improve outcomes for African-American survivors of domestic violence*. Sacramento, CA: Grant. G. Retrieved from: http://www.adp.cahwnet.gov/women/PDF/Trauma_Informed.pdf

Camacho, A., Ng, B., Bejarano, A., Simmons, A., & Chavira, D. (2012). Crisis visits and psychiatric hospitalizations among patients attending a community clinic in rural Southern California. *Journal of Community Mental Health, 48,* 133 – 7.

Cassidy, J., & Shaver, P. (2008). *Handbook of attachment: Theory, research, and clinical applications (2nd Ed.).* New York, NY: The Guliford Press.

Catalano, R., Snowden, L., Shumway, M., & Kessell, E. (2007). Unemployment and civil commitment: A Test of the intolerance hypothesis. *Aggressive Behavior, 33,* 272 – 80.

Charles, C. (2003). Skin-bleaching, self-hate, and black identity in Jamaica. *Journal of Black Studies, 33*(6), 711-728.

Chassin, L., & Handley, E. (2006). Parents and families as contexts for the development of substance abuse and substance abuse disorders. *Psychology of Addictive Behaviors,20*(2), 135-137.

Chiovitti, R. (2011). Theory of protective empowering for balancing patient safety and choices. *Nursing Ethics, 18*(1), 88 – 101.

Clarkin, J., Foelsch, P., Levy, K., Hull, J., Delaney, J., & Kernberg, O. (2001). The development of a psychoanalytic treatment for patients with borderline personality disorder: A preliminary study of behavioral change. *Journal of Personality Disorders, 15*(6), 487 – 495.

Cohen, D. (2012). Needed: Critical thinking about psychiatric medications. *Social Work in Mental Health, 7*(1-3), 42 – 61.

Connell, A., Dishion, T., Yasui, M., & Kavanaugh, K. (2007). An adaptive approach to family intervention: Linking engagement in family-centered intervention to reductions in adolescent problem behavior. *The Journal of Consulting and Clinical Psychology, 75*(4), 568 – 579.

Cook, A., Spinazzola, J., Ford, J., Lanktree, C., Blaustein, M., Cloitre, M., DeRosa, R., Hubbard, R., Kagan, R., Liautaud, J., Mallah, K., Olafson, E., & van der Kolk, B. (2008). Complex trauma in children and adolescents. *Psychiatric Annals, 35*(5), 390-398.

Corey, G. (2009). *Theory and practice of counseling and psychotherapy.* Belmont, CA: Thomson Higher Education.

Council of National Psychological Associations for the Advancement of Ethnic Minority Interests (2003, November). *Psychological treatment of ethnic minority populations.* Washington D.C. The Association of Black Psychologists. Retrieved from: http://www.apa.org/pi/oema/resources/brochures/treatment-minority.pdf

Covell, N., Weissman, E., Schell, B., McCorkle, B., Summerfelt, W., Weiden, P., & Essock, S. (2007). Distress with medication side effects among persons with severe mental illness. *Administrative Policy on Mental Health, 34,* 435 – 42.

Dattilio, F., & Bahadur, M. (2005). Cognitive-behavioral therapy with an East Indian family. *Contemporary Family Therapy, 27*(3), 367 – 382.

Davis, R., Ressler, K., Schwartz, A., Stephens, K., & Bradley, R. (2008). Treatment barriers for urban African Americans underdiagnosed with posttraumatic stress disorder. *Journal of Traumatic Stress, 21*(2), 218-222.

Deegan, P. (2007). The lived experience of using psychiatric medication in the recovery process and a shared decision-making program to support it. *Psychiatric Rehabilitation Journal, 31*(1), 62 – 9.

De la Cruz, G. (2010, December). *Traumatic impingements of immigration.* Paper presented at Winter Convocation of The Sanville Institute, Los Angeles, CA.

Del Vecchio, V., Luciano, M., Giacco, V., Vinci, u., & Fiorillo, A. (2010). Coercive measures in acute inpatient care in Italy. *European Psychiatry, 25*(3), n.p.

Diamond, D., Clarkin, J., Levine, H., Levy, K., Foelsch, P., & Yeomans, F. (1999). Borderline conditions and attachment: A preliminary report. *Psychoanalytic Inquiry, 19*, 831-884.

Diamond, D., Stovall-McClough, C., Clarkin, J., & Levy, K. (2003). Patient-therapist attachment in the treatment of borderline personality disorder. *Bulletin of the Menninger Clinic, (67)*3, 227 – 259.

Dianov, D., Maltseva, M., & Kotov, V. (2007). The system of coercive treatment (court mandated) medical measures in the Russian Federation. *BMC Psychiatry, 7*(1), n.p.

DiBonaventura, M, Gabriel, S., Dupclay, L., Gupta, S., & Kim, E. (2012). A patient perspective of the impact of medication side effects on adherence: Results of a cross-sectional nationwide survey of patients with schizophrenia. *BMC Psychiatry, 12*(20), 1 – 7.

Dmitriev, A., Vinnikova, I., Lazko, N., Ospanova, A., & Gouzenko, O. (2007). Principles of compulsory psychiatric inpatient treatment. *BMC Psychiatry, 7*(1), n.p.

Dobson, K. (2001). *Handbook of cognitive-behavioral therapies (2nd Sd.).* New York, NY: The Guliford Press.

Drake, B., & Pandley, S. (1996) Understanding the relationship between neighborhood poverty and specific types. *Child Abuse & Neglect: The International Journal, 20*(11), 1003-1018.

Druss, B., Rosenheck, R., & Stollar, M. (1999). Patient satisfaction and administrative measures as indicators of the quality of mental health care. *Journal of Psychiatric Services, 50,* 1053 – 8.

Duncan, L., & Johnson, D. (2007). Black undergraduate students attitude toward counseling and counselor preference. *College Student Journal, 41*(3), 696-719.

Dyck, A., Deschamps, M., & Taylor, J. (2005). Pharmacists' discussions of medication side effects: A Descriptive study. *Patient Education and Counseling, 56,* 21 – 7.

Eack, S., & Newhill, C. (2012). Racial disparities in mental health outcomes after psychiatric hospital discharge among individuals with severe mental illness. *Social Work Research, 36*(1), 41 – 52.

Earley, P. (2006). Crazy: A Father's search through America's mental health madness (book review). *Journal of Health Politics, Policy and Law, 32*(3), n.p.

Eastwick, Z., & Grant, A. (2005). The treatment of people with borderline personality disorder'. A cause for concern? *Mental Health Practice, 8*(7), 38 - 40.

Ebner, G., & Fraunfelder, A. (2007). An integrated concept of empowerment: A way to avoid coercive treatment. *BMC Psychiatry, 7*(1), n.p.

Ellila, H.T., Sourander, A., Valimaki, M., Warne, T., & Kaivosoja, M. (2008). The Involuntary treatment of adolescent psychiatric inpatients- A nationwide survey from Finland. *Journal of Adolescence, 31, 407 – 419.*

Erikson, E.H. (1963). *Childhood and society.* New York, NY: W.W. Norton & Company.

Erikson, E.H. (1964). *Insight and responsibility.* New York, NY: W.W. Norton & Company.

Evans, K., Kincade, E., Marbley, A., & Seem, S. (2005). Feminism and feminist-therapy: Lessons from the past and hope for the future. *Journal of Counseling & Development,*

83(3), 269 – 277.

Faasse, K. (2012). The nocebo effect: Patient expectations and medication side effects. *Postgraduate Medical Journal, 89*(1055), 540 – 6.

Fanniff, A., Otto, R., & Petrila, J. (2010). Competence to proceed in SVP commitment hearings: Irrelevant of fundamental due process right. *Behavioral Sciences and the Law, 28,* 647 – 70.

Fennell, P., & Goldstein, P. (2006). The application of civil commitment law to a case of delusional disorder: A cross-national comparison of legal approaches in the United States and the United Kingdom. *Behavioral Science and the Law, 24,* 385 – 406.

First Five Alameda County. (2011, May 5). *Mandated child abuse reporting.* Training seminar facilitated by Hernandez, R., San Leandro, CA.

Flicker, S., Turner, C., Waldron, H., Brody, J., & Ozechowski, T. (2008). Ethnic background, therapeutic alliance, and treatment retention in functional family therapy with adolescents who abuse substances. *Journal of Family Psychology, 22*(1), 167 – 170.

Freud, A. (1966). *The ego and the mechanisms of defense* (Rev. Ed.). London, UK: The Hogarth Press.

Freud, S. (2007). *Collected works of Sigmund Freud.* Charleston, SC: BiblioLife.

Garcia, J., Chang, C., Young, J., Lopez, S., & Jenkins, J. (2006). Family support predicts psychiatric medication usag e among Mexican American individuals with schizophrenia. *Social Psychiatry and Epidemiology, 41,* 624 – 31.

Garg, R., Levin, E., Urajnik, D., & Kauppi, C. (2005). Parenting style and academic achievement for East Indian and Canadian adolescents. *Journal of Comparative Family Studies, 36*(4), 653 – 661.

Gaylord-Harden, N., Ragsdale, B., Mandara, J., Richards, M., & Peterson, A. (2006). Perceived support and internalizing symptoms in African American adolescents: Self-esteem and ethnic identity. *Journal of Youth and Adolescence, 36*(1), 77-88.

Geertz, C. (1973). *The interpretation of cultures: Selected essays.* New York, NY: Basic Books.

Georgieva, I., Mulder, C., & Whittington, R. (2012). Evaluation of behavioral changes and subjective distress after exposure to coercive inpatient interventions. *BMC Psychiatry, 12*(54), 1 – 11.

Gigantesco, A., Morosini, P., 7 Bazzoni, A. (2003). Quality of psychiatric care: Validation of an instrument for measuring inpatient opinion. *International Journal for Quality in Health Care, 15*(1), 73 – 8.

Girolamo, G., Rucci, P., Gaddini, A., Picardi, A., & Santone, G. (2008). Compulsory admissions in Italy. *International Journal of Mental Health, 37*(4), 46 – 90.

Goffman, E. (1986). *Stigma: Notes on management of spoiled identity.* New York, NY: Simon & Schuster.

Goldstein, E. (1984). *Ego psychology and social work practice.* New York, NY: The Free Press.

Golier, J., Yehuda, R., Bierer, L., Mitropoulou, V., New, A., Schmeidler, J., Silverman, J., & Siever, L. (2003). The relationship of borderline personality disorder to posttraumatic stress disorder and traumatic events. *American Journal of Psychiatry, 160*(11), 2018 – 2024.

Gregory, R. (2004). Thematic stages of recovery in the treatment of borderline personality disorder. *American Journal of Psychotherapy, 58*(3), 335 - 348.

Grogan, P., & Proscio, T. (2000). *Comeback cities: A blueprint for urban neighborhood revival.* Boulder, CO: The Westview Press.

Gump, J. (2010). Reality matters: The shadow of trauma on African-American subjectivity. *Psychonalaytic Psychology, 27*(1), 42-54.

Guarda, A., Marinilli, A., Coughlin, J., Hussain, S., Haug, N., & Heinberg, L. (2007). Perceived coercion and change in perceived need for admission in patients hospitalized for eating disorders. *The American Journal of Psychiatry, 164*(1), 108 – 14.

Gurman, A., & Messer, S. (2005) *Essential psychotherapies: Theory and practice* (2nd ed.). New York, NY: The Guliford Press.

Haley, A. (1965). *The autobiography of Malcolm X.* New York, NY: Ballantine Publishing.

Hall, S (1997). *Race: The floating signifier.* Northampton, MA: The Media Education Foundation. Video Taped Lecture.

Hartman, B. (2009). Recent case developments in health law. *Journal of Law, Medicine, and Ethics,* 380 – 8.

Hartmann, H. (1958). *Ego Psychology and the problem of adaptation.* New York, NY: International Universities Press.

Hayes, S., Follete, V., & Linehan, M. (2004). *Expanding the cognitive-behavioral tradition: Mindfulness and acceptance.* New York, NY: The Guliford Press.

Henderson, C., Flood, C., Morven, L., Thornicroft, G., Sutherby, K., & Szmukler, G. (2007). Joint crisis plans reduce coercive treatment. *BMC Psychiatry, 7*91), n.p.

Henderson, C., Greenbaum, P., Dakof, G., & Liddle, H. (2010). Effectiveness of multidimensional family therapy with higher severity substance-abusing adolescents: Report from two randomized controlled trials. *Journal of Consulting and Clinical Psychology, 78*(6), 885 – 897.

Herman, J. (1996). *Trauma and recovery: The aftermath of violence -from domestic abuse to political terror.* New York, NY: Basic Books.

Herron, W., Guido, S., & Kantor, R. (1965). Relationships among ego strength measures. *Journal of Clinical Psychology, 21*(4), 403-404.

Holm, J., Brixen, K., Andries, A., Horder, K., & Stoving, R. (2012). Reflections on involuntary treatment in the prevention of fatal anorexia nervosa: A review of five cases. *International Journal of Eating Disorders, 45*(1), 93 – 100.

Hopko, D., Averill, P., Cowan, K., & Shah, N. (2002). Self-reported and treatment outcome among non-offending involuntary inpatients. *Journal of Forensic Psychiatry, 13*(1), 88 – 106.

Huber, C., Schottle, D., Lambert, M., Hottenrott, B., Agorastos, A., Naber, D., & Schroeder, K. (2012). Brief Psychiatric Rating Scale (BPRS) – excited component (BPRS-EC) and neuropsychological dysfunction predict aggression, suicidality, and involuntary treatment in first-episode psychosis. *Schizophrenia Research, 134,* 273 – 278.

Hughes, D. (2006). *Building the bonds of attachment: Awakening love in deeply troubled children* (2nd ed.). Lanham, MD: Rowman and Littlefield Publishers, Inc.

Hughes, D. (2007). *Attachment-focused family therapy.* W.W. Norton & Co.: New York, NY.

Hughes, R., Hayward, M., & Finlay, W. (2009). Patients perceptions of the impact of involuntary inpatient care on self, relationships, and recovery. *Journal of Mental Health, 18*(2), 152 – 60.

Hugo, M. (1999). Comparative efficiency ratings between public and private acute inpatient facilities. *Australian and New Zealand Journal of Psychiatry, 34,* 651 – 7.

Hustoft, K., Larsen, T., Auestad, B., Joa, I., Johannessen, J., & Ruud, T. (2013). Predictors of involuntary hospitalizations to acute psychiatry. *International Journal of Law and Psychiatry, 36,* 136-143.

Ilgen, M., Tiet, Q., & Finney, J. (2006). Quality of therapeutic relationship associated with better treatment outcomes. *The Brown University Digest of Addiction Theory & Application, 25*(9), 1-7.

Institute for Safe Medication Practice (2014). Cultural diversity and medication safety. Retrieved from www.ismp.org/newsletters/acutecare/articles/20030904.asp

Iverson, K., Hoyer, G., Sexton, H. (2009). Rates for civil commitment to psychiatric hospitals in Norway. Are registry data accurate? *Nordic Journal of Psychiatry, 63*(4), 301 – 7.

Jarrett, M., Bowers, L., & Simpson, A. (2008). Coerced medication in psychiatric inpatient care: Literature review. *Journal of Advanced Nursing, 64*(6), 538 – 48.

Johnson, R. (2002). Racial identity from an African-American perspective. *Journal of Cultural Diversity, Fall 2002*, n.p.

Jones, E. (1978). Black-white personality differences: Another look. *Journal of Personality Assessment, 42*(3), 244-252.

Jones, E. (1982). Psychotherapists' impressions of treatment outcome as a function of race. *Journal of Clinical Psychology, 38*(4), 722-731.

Jones, E. (1982). *Minority mental health.* Essex, UK: Abbey Publishing.

Jones, E. (1984). Some reflections on the black patient and psychotherapy. *Clinical Psychologist,* 37(2), 62-65.

Jones, M., & Jones, A. (2007). Delivering the choice agenda as a framework to manage adverse effects: A Mental health nurse perspective on prescribing medication. *Journal of Psychiatric and Mental Health Nursing, 14,* 418 – 23.

Kilpatrick, D., Acierno, R., Saunders, B., Resnick, H., Best, C., & Schnurr, P. (2000). Risk factors for adolescent substance abuse and dependence: Data from a national sample. *Journal of Consulting and Clinical Psychology, 68*(1), 19 – 30.

Kimmerling, R., Ouimette, P., & Wolfe, J. (2002). *Gender and PTSD.* New York, NY: The Guliford Press.

Kjellen, L. (2007). Policies regarding coercive care in Swedish child and adolescent psychiatry. *BMC Psychiatry, 7*(1), n.p.

Knifton, L., Gervais, M., Newbigging, K., Mirza, N., Quinn, N., Wilson, W., & Hunkins Hutchison, H. (2010). Community conversation: Addressing mental health stigma with ethnic minority communities. *Journal of Social Psychiatry and Epidemiology, 45,* p. 497 – 504.

Kozol, J. (2005). *The shame of the nation: The restoration of apartheid schooling in America.* New York: Three Rivers Press.

Krawitz, R., Jackson, W., Allen, R., Connell, A., Argyle, N., Bensemann, C., & Mileshkin, C. (2004). Professionally indicated short-term risk-taking in the treatment of borderline personality disorder. *Australasian Psychiatry, 12*(1), 11 – 17.

Krawitz, R., & Watson, C. (2000) Borderline personality disorder: Foundations of treatment. *Australian Social Work, 56*(2), 175 – 177.

Kundu, S., Adams, G. (2005). Identity formation, individuality, and connectedness in East Indian and non East Indian female Canadian emerging adults. *Identity: An International Journal of Theory and Research, 5*(3), 247 – 260.

Kwak, K., & Berry, J. (2001). Generational differences in acculturation among Asian families in Canada: A comparison of Vietnamese, Korean, and East-Indian groups. *International Journal of Psychology, 36*(3), 152 – 162.

Lebel, J. (2007). Regulatory, clinical, and educational approaches to eliminating restraint and seclusion. *BMC Psychiatry, 7*(1), n.p.

Liddle, H., Rowe, C., Dakof, G., & Henderson, C. (2009). Multidimensional family therapy for young adolescent substance abuse: Twelve-month outcomes of a randomized controlled trial. *Journal of Consulting and Clinical Psychology, 77*(1), 12 – 25.

Lieberman, A., & Van Horn, P. (2008). *Psychotherapy with infants and young children: Repairing the effects of stress and trauma on early attachment.* New York, NY: The Guliford Press.

Lindellus, B. (2012). Involuntary treatment in Swedish psychiatry. *European Psychiatry, 27*(2,3), n.p.

Linehan, M., Armstrong, H., Suarez, A., Allmon, D., & Heard, H. (1991). Cognitive–behavioral treatment of chronically parasuicidal borderline patients. *Archives of General Psychiatry, 48*(12), 971–974.

Linehan, M. (1993). *Cognitive-behavioral treatment of borderline personality disorder.* New York, NY: The Guliford Press.

Linehan, M. (1993). *Skills training manual for treating borderline personality disorder.* New York, NY: The Guliford Press.

Livesley, J (2005). Progress in the treatment of borderline personality disorder. *The Canadian Journal of Psychiatry. 50*(8), 433 – 434.

Logan, S. (2001). *The black family: Strengths, self-help, and positive change* (2nd ed.). Oxford, UK: The Westview Press.

Lum, D. (2003). *Social work practice and people of color* (5th ed.). Florence, KY: Wadsworth Publishing.

Lyons, J., O'Mahoney, M., Miller, S., Neme, J., Kabat, J., & Miller, F. (1997). Predicting readmission to the psychiatric hospital in a managed care environment: Implications for quality indicators. *American Journal of Psychiatry, 154*(3), 337 – 40.

Macy, R., Behar, L., Paulson, R., Delman, J., Schmid, L., & Smith, S. (2004). Community based, acute posttraumatic stress-management: A description and evaluation of a psychosocial-intervention continuum. *Harvard Review of Psychiatry, 12*(4), 217-228.

Main, M., & Solomon, J. (1986). Discovery of an insecure disorganized/disoriented attachment pattern: Procedures, findings and implications for classification of behaviour. In M.W. Yogman & T.B. Brazelton, *Affective development in infancy.* 95-124. Norwood, NJ: Ablex Publishing Corporation.

Markstrom, C., & Hunter, C.L. (1999). The roles of ethnic and ideological identity in predicting fidelity in African American and European American adolescents. *Child Study Journal, 29*(1), 23-39.

Markstrom, C., & Kalmanir, H. (2001) Linkages between the psychosocial stages of identity and intimacy and the ego strengths of fidelity and love. *Journal of Theory and Research, 1*(2), 179-196.

Markstrom, C., Sabino, V., Turner, B., & Berman, R. (1997). The psychosocial inventory of ego strengths: Development and validation of a new Eriksonian measure. *Journal of Youth and Adolescence, 26*(6), 705-733.

Markstrom, C., & Marshall, S. (2007). The psychosocial inventory of ego strengths: Examination of theory and psychometric properties. *Journal of Adolescence, 20*(1), 63-79.

Mason, T., Worsley, Q., & Coyle, D. (2010). Forensic multidisciplinary perspectives on Tarasoff liability: A vignette study. *The Journal of Forensic Psychiatry & Psychology, 21*(4), 549 – 554.

McCart, M., Henggeler, S., Chapman, J., & Cunningham, P. (2012). System-level effects of integrating a promising treatment into juvenile drug courts. *Journal of Substance Abuse Treatment, 43,* 231 – 43.

McEwann, S., de Man, A., & Simpson-Housley, P. (2005). Acquaintance rape, ego identity achievement, and locus of control. *Social Behavior & Personality, 33*(6), 567-592.

McEwann, S., de Man, A., & Simpson-Housley, P. (2002). Ego-identity achievement and perception of risk in intimacy in survivors of stranger and acquaintance rape. *Sex Roles: A Journal of Research, 47*(5, 6), 281-287.

McGoldrick, M, & Hardy, K. (2009). *Re-envisioning family therapy: Race, culture, and gender in clinical practice* (2nd ed.). New York, NY: The Guliford Press.

McRee, N., and Drapela, L. (2012). The Timing and accumulation of judicial sanctions among drug court clients. *Journal of Crime & Delinquency, 58*(6), 911 – 931.

Medora, N., Larson, J., & Dave, P. (2003). Attitudes of East-Indian college students toward family strengths. *Journal of Comparative Family Studies, 31*(4), 407 – 425.

McNally, RJ. (2007). Betrayal trauma theory: A critical appraisal. *Journal of Memory, 15*(3), 280-294.

Meehan, T., Stedman, T., & Wallace, J. (2011). Consumer strategies for coping with antipsychotic medication side effects. *The Royal Australian and New Zealand College of Psychiatrists, 19*(1), 74 – 7.

Mendel, R., Traut-Mattausch, E., Frey, D., Buhner, M., Berthele, A., Kissling, W., & Hamann, J. (2011). Do physicians' recommendations pull patients away from their preferred treatment options? *Health Expectations, 15,* 23 – 31.

Mental Health Weekly (1999). *Array of involuntary treatment bills in N.Y. take opposing approaches, 9*(23), n.p.

Michalopoulos, L, & Boyd, R.C. (2009, June). *Trauma, depression, and kinship support among Urban African-American women.* Paper presented at the annual meeting of the SCRA Biennial meeting at Montclair State University, Montclair, NJ. Retrieved from: http://www.allacademic.com/meta/p_mla_apa_research_citation/3/0/1/3/7/p301378_index.html

Mitchell, S., & Black, M. (1995). *Freud and beyond.* New York, NY: Basic Books.

Moffat, J., Sass, B., McKenzie, K., & Bhui, K. (2009). Improving pathways into mental health care for black and ethnic minority groups: A systematic review of the grey literature. *International Review of Psychiatry, 21*(5), 439 – 449.

Monahan, J. (1993). Limiting therapist exposure to Tarasoff liability: Guidelines for risk containment. *American Psychologist, 48*(3), 242 – 50.

Morrison, P., Meehan, T., Gaskill, D., Lunney, P., & Collings, P. (2000). Enhancing case managers' skills in the assessment and management of antipsychotic medication side effects. *Australian and New Zealand Journal of Psychiatry, 34,* 814 – 21.

Mrad, D. (2009). The pre-sell medication controversy: Restoring competency at the end of the 20th century. *Journal of Psychiatry & Law, 37,* 341 – 72.

Mui, C. (2005). A Feminist-Sartrean approach to understanding rape trauma. *Sartre Studies International, An Interdisciplinary Journal of Existentialism and Contemporary Culture, 11*(1, 2), 153-165.

Munetz, M., & Frese, F. (2001). Getting ready for recovery: Reconciling mandatory treatment with the recovery vision. *Psychiatric Rehabilitation Journal, 25*(1), 35 – 41.

N. A. (1984). Mental patients – involuntary treatment – Rogers v. Commissioner of the Department of Mental Health. *American Journal of Law & Medicine, 9*(4), n.p.

N. A. (1985). Civil commitment – involuntary treatment – *People v. Medina. American Journal of Law & Medicine, 11*(3), n.p.

N. A. (1986). Compulsory treatment of the mentally ill. *British Medical Journal (Clinical Research Journal), 292*(6524), 888 – 9.

Nace, E., Birkmayer, F., Sullivan, M., Galanter, M., Fromson, J., Frances, R., Levin, F., Lewis, C., Suchinsky, R., Tamerin, J., & Westermeyer, J. (2007). Socially sanctioned coercion mechanisms for addiction treatment. *The American Journal on Addictions, 16,* 15 – 23.

Natrajan, R., Karuppaswamy, N., Thomas, V., & Ramadoss, K. (2005). Adaptation of two family therapy training instruments to culturally suit the Indian context. *Contemporary Family Therapy, 23*(3), 415 – 434.

Neacsiu, A., Rizvi, S., & Linehan, M. (2010). Dialectical behavior therapy skills use as a mediator and outcome of treatment for borderline personality disorder. *Behavior Research and Therapy, 48*(9), 832 - 839.

Nelson, J. (2005). *Seeing through tears.* New York, NY: Brunner-Routledge.

Newsletter of the center: Posttraumatic disorders program. (1998). *Trauma and the African American experience* [*3*(2)]. Washington, D.C.: Reese, C.

Olsen, D. (2003). Influence and coercion: Relational and rights-based ethical approaches to forced psychiatric treatment. *Journal of Psychiatric and Mental Health Nursing, 10,* 705 – 12.

Opsal, A., Kristensen, O., Larsen, T., Syversen, G., Rudshaug, E., Gerdner, A., & Clausen, T. (2013). Factors associated with involuntary admissions among patients with substance abuse disorders and comorbidity: A cross-sectional study. *BMC Health Services Research, 13*(57), 1-8.

Oumaya, M., Friedman, S., Pham, A., Abou Abdallah, T., Guelfi, J.D., Roullin, F. (2008). Borderline personality disorder, self-mutilation and suicide: Literature review. *Encephale, 34*(5), 452 – 458.

Parham, T., White, J., & Ajamu, A. (1999). *The psychology of blacks: An African centered perspective* (3rd ed.). Upper Saddle River, NJ: Prentice Hall.

Patterson, C.H. (1959). *Counseling and psychotherapy: Theory and practice.* New York, NY: Harper & Row.

Phillip, C., Mahalingam, R., & Sellers, R. (2010). Understanding East Indians' attitudes toward African Americans: Do mainstream prejudicial attitudes transfer to immigrants? *Journal of Ethnic and Migration Studies, 36*(4), 651 – 671.

Phillips, M. (2013). Can China's new mental health law substantially reduce the burden of illness attributable to mental disorders? *American Journal of Psychiatry, 381,* 1964 – 66.

Phillips, M., Chen, H., Diesfeld, K., Zie, B., Cheng, H., Mellsop, G., & Liu, X. (2013). China's new mental health law: Reframing involuntary treatment. *American Journal of Psychiatry, 170*(6), 588 – 91.

Pinta, E. (2010). *Tarasoff* duties in prison: Community standards with certain twists. *Psychiatric Quarterly, 81,* 177 – 182. DOI: 10.1007/s11126-010-9127-1.

Poulsen, S. (2009). East Indian families raising ABCD adolescents: Cultural and generational challenges. *The Family Journal, 17*(2), 168 – 174.

Prochaska, J. (1979). *Systems of psychotherapy: A transtheoretical analysis.* Homewood, IL: Dorsey Press.

Public Broadcasting System (2009, April 20). Re: Minorities and Mental Health. [Online posting] Retrieved from: http://www.pbs.org/wnet/cryforhelp/episodes/resources minorities-and-mental-health/23/

Reamer, F., & Kelly, M. (1990). Should competence be coerced? *Hastings Center Report, 20*(4), n.p.

Regan, K. (2010). Trauma informed care on an inpatient pediatric psychiatric unit and the emergence of ethical dilemmas as nurses evolved their practice. *Issues in Mental Health Nursing, 31,* 216 – 222.

Ries, R., Yuodelis-Flores, C., Roy-Byrne, P., Nilssen, O., and Russo, J. (2009). Addiction and suicidal behavior in acute psychiatric inpatients. *Comprehensive Psychiatry, 50,* 93-99.

Robinson, L. (1995). *Psychology for social workers: Black perspectives.* New York, NY: Brunner-Routledge.

Rodrigues, T., Castro, L., Pereira, J., & Pereira, H. (2009). Acute inpatient units' old challenges: Compulsory versus voluntary treatment. *European Psychiatry, 24*(1), n.p.

Roe, D., Goldblatt, H., Bloush-Klienman, V., SWarbick, M., & Davidson, L. (2009). Why and how people decide to stop taking psychiatric medication: Exploring the subjective process of choice. *Psychiatric Rehabilitation Journal, 33*(1), 38 – 46.

Rowe, C., & Isaac, D. (1991). *Empathic attunement: The "technique" of psychoanalytic self psychology.* Northvale, NJ: Jason Aronson Publishers Inc.

Ruggeri, M. (1994). Patients' and relatives' satisfaction with psychiatric services: The State of the art and ites measurement. *Social Psychiatry Research and Epidemiology, 29,* 212 – 27.

Ruiz, P., Strain, E., Langford, J. (2007). *The Substance abuse handbook.* Lippincott Williams & Wilkins: Philadelphia, PA.

Ryan, W. (1971). *Blaming the victim.* New York, NY: Pantheon Books.

Rydelius, P. (2007). Inpatient and emergency child and adolescent psychiatry units in Sweden do not use restraint and seclusion: What we have learned. *BMC Psychiatry, 7*(1), n.p.

Rymaszewska, J. (2007). Patients' subjective quality of life during involuntary treatment in psychiatric hospitals. *BMC Psychiatry, 7,* 1.

Sable, P. (2000). *Attachment and adult psychotherapy.* Lanham, MD: Rowman & Littlefield Publishers, Inc.

Sachsse, U., Vogel, C., & Leichsenring, D. (2006). Results of psychodynamically oriented trauma–focused inpatient treatment for women with complex posttraumatic stress disorder (PTSD) and borderline personality disorder (BPD). *The Bulletin of the Menninger Clinic: A Journal for the Mental Health Professions. 70*(2), 125 – 144.

Saigh, P., Yasik, A., Oberfield, R., & Halamandaris, P. (2008). The self-concept of traumatized children and adolescents with or without PTSD. *Behaviour Research and Therapy, 46*(10), 1181-1186.

Saleeby, D. (2009). *The strengths perspective in social work practice.* Boston, MA: Allyn & Bacon.

Salize, H.J., & Dressing, H. (2011). Approaches to civil commitment in psychiatry in Europe. *Journal of Psychiatry, 22*(4), 113 – 20.

Schiller, J. (2009, October). *Contemporary psychoanalytic perspective on a case presentation: "Finding Lisa."* Paper presented at the Fall Convocation of The Sanville Institute, Berkeley, CA.

Schnittker, J. (2003). Misgivings of medicine? African Americans' skepticism of psychiatric medication. *Journal of Health and Social Behavior, 44,* 506 – 24.

Schnopp, R. (2006). Involuntary treatment and competence to proceed in the criminal process: Capital and noncapital cases. *Behavioral Sciences and the Law, 24,* 495 – 528.

Schore, A. (2003). *Affect dysregulation and disorders of the self.* New York, NY: W.W. Norton & Company.

Schore, A., & Schore, J. (2008). Modern attachment theory: The central role of affect regulation in development and treatment. *Clinical social work journal*, 36(1), 9-20.

Scott, Williams, & Beck. (1995). *Cognitive therapy in clinical practice: An illustrative casebook.* New York, NY: Brunner-Routledge.

Segal, S., & Burgess, P. (2008). Use of community treatment orders to prevent psychiatric hospitalization. *Australian and New Zealand Journal of Psychiatry, 42,* 732 – 9.

Sharpe, T. (2010, n.m.). *Working with African-American families who have experienced trauma.* Paper presented at University of Maryland School of Social Work, College Park MD.

Shelef, K., Diamond, Ga., Diamond, Gu., & Liddle, H. (2005). Adolescent and parent alliance and treatment outcome in multidimensional family therapy. *Journal of Consulting and Clinical Psychology, 73*(4), 689 – 698.

Shybut, J. (2006). Internal vs. external control, time perspective, and delay of gratification of high and low ego strength groups. *Journal of Clinical Psychology, 26*(4), 430-431.

Sindel, P. (1991). Fourteenth amendment – The Right to refuse antipsychotic drugs masked by prison bars. *Journal of Criminal Law and Criminology, 81*(4), 951 – 81.

Siponen, U., Valimaki, M., Kaivosoja, M., Marttunen, M., & Kaltiala-Heino, R. (2007). Increase in involuntary psychiatric treatment and child welfare placements in Finald 1996 – 2003. *Journal of Social Psychiatry and Psychiatric Epidemiology, 42,* 146 – 152.

Skeem, J., Silver, E., Aippelbaum, P., & Tiemann, J. (2006). Suicide-related behavior after psychiatric hospital discharge: Implications for risk assessment and management. *Behavioral Sciences and the Law, 24,* 731 – 46.

Smith, G. (2003). Essay book review. *Journal of Family Therapy, 14*(4), 213 – 222.

Sodertstrom, K., & Skarderud, F. (2009). *Minding the Baby:* Mentalization-based treatment in Families with parental substance use disorder: Theoretical framework. *Nordic Psychology, 61*(3), 47 – 65.

Soloman, M., & Siegel, D. (2003). *Healing trauma: Attachment, mind, body, and brain.* New York, NY: W. W. Norton & Company.

Spellecy, R. (2007). Psychiatric outpatient commitment: One tool along a continuum. *The American Journal of Bioethics, 7*(11), 45 – 7.

Sperry (1995). *Handbook of diagnosis and treatment of DSM-IV personality disorders* (1st ed.). London, UK: Brunner-Routledge.

Spinazzola, J., Blaustein, M., & Van Der Kolk, B. (2005). Posttraumatic stress disorder treatment outcome research: The study of unrepresentative samples? *Journal of Traumatic Stress, 18*(5), 425-436.

Steinert, T. (2007). Epidemiology of inpatient violence and coercive measures. *BMC Psychiatry, 7*(1), n.p.

Stellwagen, K., & Kerig, P. (2010). Relating callous-emotional traits to physically restrictive treatment measures among child psychiatric inpatients. *Journal of Child and Family Studies, 19*, 588 – 95.

Stewart, C., Cockburn, T., Madden, B., Callaghan, S., & Ryan, C. (2012). Leave to intervene in cases of gender identity disorder; Normative causation; Financial harms and involuntary treatment; and the right to be protected from suicide. *Bioethical Inquiry, 9*, 235-242.

Stewert, E., & Simons, R. (2006). Structure and culture in African American adolescent violence: A partial test of "the cods of the streets" thesis. *Justice Quarterly, 23*(1), 1-33.

Stone, A., & Merlo, L. (2012). Psychiatric medication-seeking beliefs and behaviors among college students. *The American Journal of Drug and Alcohol Abuse, 38*(4), 314 – 21.

Stone, D., Patton, B., & Heen, S. (2000). *Difficult conversations: How to discuss what matters most.* New York, NY: Penguin Books.

Street, A., Gibson, L., & Holohan, D. (2005). Impact of traumatic events, trauma-related guilt, and avoidant coping strategies on PTSD symptoms in female survivors of domestic violence. *Journal of Traumatic Stress, 18*(3), 245-252.

Sue, D.W (2000). *Overcoming personal racism: What can I do?* Microfilmed lecture recorded at Microtraining Associate Films, Boston, MA.

Sue, D.W. & Sue. D. (2008) Counseling the culturally diverse: Theory and practice (5th ed.) Hoboken, NJ: John Wiley & Sons, Inc.

Svindseth, M., Nottestad, J., & Dahl, A. (2013). Perceived humiliation during admission to a psychiatric emergency service and its relation to socio-demography and psychopathology. *BMC Psychiatry, 13*, 1 – 8.

Swanson, J., Swartz, M., Elbogen, E., Wagner, R., & Burns, B. (2003). Effects of involuntary outpatient commitment on subjective quality of life in persons with severe mental illness. *Behavioral Sciences and the Law, 21*, 473 – 91.

Tataru, N., & Dicker, A. (2009). Geriatric psychiatry and human rights in Romania – involuntary treatment. *European Psychiatry, 24*(1), n.p.

Taube, D. (2013). Mandated reporting: Tarasoff. Power point lecture at Alliant International University, 10/23/13.

Taube, D. (2013b). Substantive patients rights and Lanterman-Petris-Short. Power point lecture at Alliant International University, 11/25/13.

Tolmac, J., & Hodes, M. (2004). Ethnic variation among psychiatric in-patients with Psychotic disorders. *Journal of British Psychiatry*, 184, 428 – 31.

Tolou-Shams, M., Hadley, W., Conrad, S., & Brown, L. (2012). The Role of family affect in juvenile court offenders substance abuse and HIV risk. *Journal of Child and Family Studies, 21*, 449 – 456.

Townsend, L. (2009). How effective are interventions to enhance adherence to psychiatric medications? Practice implications for social workers working with adults diagnosed with severe mental illness. *Journal of Health and Human Behavior in the Social Environment, 19*, 512 – 30.

Tuohimäki, C., Kaltiala-Heino, R., Korkeila, J., Tuori, T., Lehtinen, V., & Joukamaa, M. (2003). The Use of harmful to others criteria for involuntary hospitalization in Finland.

European Journal of Health Law, 10(2), 183 – 199. DOI: 10.1163/092902703769681614.

Tucker, J. (2007, August 26). Children who survive urban warfare suffer from PTSD. *The San Francisco Chronicle*. pp. A-1.

Turbott, J. (2004). Treatment of borderline personality disorder. *Australasian Psychiatry, 12*(3), 259.

Usahacharoenporn, P. (2011). E.P. vs. Alaska Psychiatric Institutute: The Evolution of involuntary civil commitment from treatment to punishment. *Alaska Law Review, 28*(189), 1 -11.

Valliant, G. (1993). *The wisdom of the ego*. Cambridge, MA: Harvard University Press.

Van der Kolk, B., Pelcovitz, D., Roth, S., Mandel, F., McFarlane, A., & Herman, J. (1996). Dissociation, affect dysregulation, and somatization: The complexity of adaptation to trauma. *American Journal of Psychiatry, 153*(7), 83-93.

Van der Kolk, B., Roth, S., Pelcovitz, D., Sunday, S., & Spinazzola, J. (2005). Disorders of extreme stress: The empirical foundation of a complex adaptation to trauma. *Journal of Traumatic Stress, 18*(5), 389-399.

Vuckovich, P., & Artinian, B. (2005). Justifying Coercion. *Nursing Ethics, 12*(4), 370 – 9.

Wachtel, P. (1993). *Therapeutic communication: Knowing what to say when*. New York, NY: The Guliford Press.

Wachtel, P., & Messer, S. (1997). *Theories of psychotherapy: Origins and evolution*.

Washington, DC: American Psychological Association.

Waites, C. (2004). *Social work practice with African-American families: An intergenerational perspective*. New York, NY: Brunner-Routledge.

Walker, C. (2004). Modernity in black: Dubois and the (re) construction of black identity in the souls of black folk. *Philosophia Africana, 7*(1), 83-93.

Wallin, D. (2007). *Attachment in psychotherapy*. New York, NY: The Guliford Press.

Wallsten, T., & Kjellen. (2007). Patients' experience of coercive treatment and coercive measures in psychiatric care. *BMC Psychiatry, 7*(1), n.p.

Watson, T., Bowers, B., & Anderson, A. (2000). Involuntary treatment of eating disorders. *The American Journal of Psychiatry, 157*(11) , 1806-1810.

Weber, D., & Reynolds, C. (2004). Clinical perspectives on neurobiological effects of trauma. *Neuropsychological Review, 14*(2), 155 – 129.

Weinberg, M. K., & Tronick, E. (1994). Beyond the face: An empirical study of infant affective configurations of facial, vocal, gestural, and regulatory behaviors. *Journal of Child Development, 65*(5), 1503-1515.

White, M., & Epston, D. (1990). *Narrative means to therapeutic ends*. New York, NY: W.W. Norton & Company.

Wilson, W. (2009). *More than just race: Being black and poor in the inner city*. New York, NY: W.W. Norton & Company.

Winkler, D., Naderi-Heiden, A., Strnad, A., Pjrek, E., Scharfeetter, J., Kasper, S., & Frey, R. (2011). Intensive care in psychiatry. *European Psychiatry, 26,* 260 – 4.

World Bank (2013). Population Growth (annual%). Retrieved from: www.data.worldbank.org/indicator/SP.POP.GROW?page=2

Xiao, J., Preston, N., & Kisely, S. (2004). What determines compulsory community treatment? A logistic regression analysis using linked mental health and offender databases. *Australian and New Zealand Journal of Psychiatry, 38,* 613 – 18.

Young, A. (2004). *The minds of marginalized black men.* Princeton, NJ: Princeton University Press.

Zanarini, M., Frankenburg, F., Dubo, E., Sickel, A., Trikha, A., Levin, A., & Reynolds, V. (1998). Axis I comorbidity of borderline personality disorder. *The American Journal of Psychiatry, 155*(12), 1733 – 1739.

Zeller, S. (2010). Treatment of psychiatric patients in emergency settings. *Primary Psychiatry, 17*(6), 41 – 47.

Zenner, G., & Munk, I. (2007). Absconding of patients on acute psychiatric wards. *BMC Psychiatry, 7*(1), n.p.

Zikmund-Fisher, B. (2008). Alternate methods of framing information about medication side effects: Incremental risk versus total risk of occurrence. *Journal of Health Communications, 13,* 107 – 24.

Zinzow, H., Ruqqiero, K., Hanson, R., Smith, D., Saunders, B., & Kilpatrick, D. (2009). Witnessed community and parental violence in relation to substance abuse and delinquency in a national sample of adolescents. *The Journal of Traumatic Stress, 22*(6), 525 – 533.

Zucker, M., Spinazzola, J., Blaustein, M., & Van Der Kolk, B. (2006). Dissociative symptomology in posttraumatic stress disorder and disorders of extreme stress. *Journal of Trauma and Dissociation, 7*(1), 19-31.

AUTHORS' CONTACT INFORMATION

Graham Danzer, PsyD Trainee ASW PPSC MRAS
Alliant International University,
California School for Professional Psychology, CA, US
E-mail: gemineyeX3@hotmail.com

Simon Ferber, PsyD Trainee
(co-author, Chapter 4)
Alliant International University,
California School for Professional Psychology, CA, US

INDEX

B

C

D

E

F

G

N

O

P

Q

R

S

T

U

V

W

Y